ADVANCED TECHNOLOGY FOR DELIVERING THERAPEUTICS

Edited by **Sabyasachi Maiti** and **Kalyan Kumar Sen**

Advanced Technology for Delivering Therapeutics
http://dx.doi.org/10.5772/62564
Edited by Sabyasachi Maiti and Kalyan Kumar Sen

Contributors

Kazuo Shimizu, Jaroslav Kristof, Jinxiang Xi, Xiuhua Si, Asadullah Madni, Nayab Tahir, Mubashar Rehman, Ahmad Raza, Muhammad Ahmad Mahmood, Muhammad Imran Khan, Prince Muhammad Kashif, Mohsin Kazi, S Lakshmana Prabu, Rathinasabapathy Thirumurugan, Suriyaprakash Tnk, K Ruckmani, Pedro Barata, Ana Rita Fernandes, Ana Oliveira, Jorge Pereira, Sabyasachi Maiti

Published by InTech
Janeza Trdine 9, 51000 Rijeka, Croatia

Publishing Process Manager Diana Olloni
Technical Editor SPi Global
Cover InTech Design team

First published May, 2017
Printed in Croatia
Legal deposit, Croatia: National and University Library in Zagreb

Additional hard copies can be obtained from orders@intechopen.com

Advanced Technology for Delivering Therapeutics, Edited by Sabyasachi Maiti and Kalyan Kumar Sen
p. cm.
Print ISBN 978-953-51-3121-2
Online ISBN 978-953-51-3122-9

For EU product safety concerns:
IN TECH d.o.o., Prolaz Marije Krucifikse Kozulić 3, 51000 Rijeka, Croatia,
info@intechopen.com or visit our website at intechopen.com.

Meet the editors

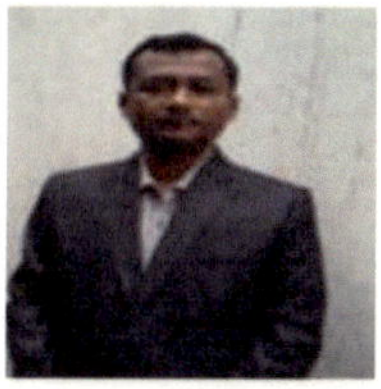

Sabyasachi Maiti is an M. Pharm, Ph D from Jadavpur University, Kolkata, India. Currently, he is working as Professor at the Department of Pharmaceutics, Gupta College of Technological Sciences, Asansol under Maulana Abul Kalam Azad University of Technology, Kolkata, India. He is working on biomaterials and their derivatives in designing controlled release drug delivery systems. He has authored and co-authored more than 50 research publications and 20 book chapters. He has guided one doctoral and more than 20 Master's thesis. He has also served as a reviewer for various journals of international repute. He has received grants for organizing seminars as well as for research projects from national funding agencies. He is a life member of IPA, Indian Chemical Society and APTI.

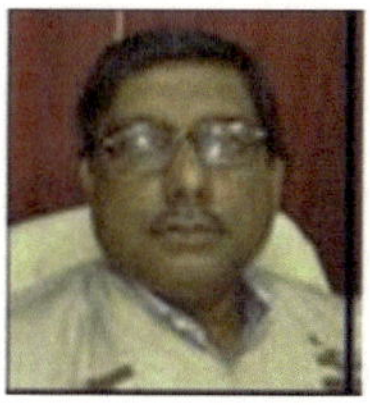

Dr. Kalyan Kumar Sen is an M.Pharm, PhD from Jadavpur University, Kolkata, India. He has twenty-nine years work experience in the field of pharmacy. He is presently working as Principal, Gupta College of Technological Sciences, Asansol, India. He is life member of professional bodies like the Association of Pharmaceutical Teachers of India (APTI), Indian Society for Technical Education (ISTE) and Indian Science Congress Association. He has successfully guided more than forty postgraduate students and two PhD students. He has several publications in international and national peer reviewed journals. He has edited one book published by CRC Press, UK and contributed several book chapters. His area of research interest is design of nanoparticulate drug delivery and vaccine delivery system.

Contents

Preface

The drug delivery system (DDS) translates drug discovery and pharmacological research into clinical practice. The treatment of acute diseases or chronic illness is accomplished by delivery of drugs to patients using various pharmaceutical dosage forms. The conventional dosage forms, which provide a prompt release of a drug, are the major pharmaceutical products in the markets. The use of conventional dosage forms results in significant fluctuations in plasma drug levels and therefore, multiple dosing has been suggested to maintain plasma drug concentration for effective treatment.

To achieve as well as to maintain the drug concentration within the therapeutically effective range and prevent fluctuations in plasma drug levels, new DDS has emerged. The science and technology responsible for the development of new DDS have been the focus of a great deal of attention in both industrial and academic laboratories. Because novel DDS can control the rate of drug release, sustain the duration of therapeutic activity, and/or target the drug to a tissue, they are expected to revolutionize the method of medication with a number of potential therapeutic benefits including patient compliance and reduced side effects.

The current focus in delivery system design is shifting to a 'smart drug' paradigm, in which increased efficacy, stability against biochemical degradation and decreased toxicity are the motivating factors. This could be achieved with targeted nanoparticles, where repertoires of targets and a series of drugs could yield new generations of highly specific therapeutic agents. The ultimate goal of nanodrug delivery systems is to develop clinically useful formulations for treating diseases. In cases where remote organs or cells (such as cells within solid tumors) are the targets, there is still a need to find ways to navigate nanoparticles through the labyrinth to the target site while avoiding clearance. Toward that goal, there have been reports of using hydrophilic coatings to achieve enhanced circulation time. Even with breakthroughs in the engineering of long-circulating nanoparticles, there is still the additional challenge of understanding and achieving the dosing that delivers consistent pharmacokinetics. In order to transform nanotechnologies from basic research into clinical products, it is important to understand how the biodistribution of NPs, which is primarily governed by their ability to negotiate biological barriers, affects the body's complex biological network, as well as mass transport across compartmental boundaries in the body. Experts from different disciplines are putting their efforts together to translate novel laboratory innovation into commercially viable medical products. Optimizing the integration of nanomaterials into drug delivery systems may result in a better understanding of the interactions of nanomaterials with biological systems, which will facilitate better engineering of their properties specific to biomedical applications. The development of such drug carriers will require a greater understanding of both the surface chemistry of nanomaterials and the interaction chemistry of these nanomaterials with biological systems. Understanding both the benefits and the risks of these new nanotechnology applications will be essential to good decision-making for drug developers, regulators and ultimately the consumers and patients who will be the beneficiaries of new drug delivery technologies. Advances in this area have allowed some nanomedicines in the market to achieve desirable pharmacokinetic properties, reduce toxicity and improve patient compliance, as well as clinical outcomes. In addition, several other experimental drug delivery systems have shown exciting signs of promise, including those composed of biodegradable polymers. It is not possible to cover all the innovative ideas in this book. This book is designed to fulfill a perceived need to provide a comprehensive picture of some novel drug delivery systems. To accomplish this task, we have organized the book in the following manner. The book starts with an introductory chapter to gain preliminary understanding on the topics and explain significance of the content covered in this book. In recent days, nanotechnology represents a powerful tool in the field of medicine to combat a plethora of diseases. Thus, the nanoscale structures (< 1000 nm) enable targeted delivery to the site of action resulting in higher therapeutic efficacy and are therefore extensively used as therapeutic carriers. Gene therapy is a medical intervention that uses genes for the treatment or prevention of disease. The biocompatible nanoparticles have been investigated for gene therapy to overcome the disadvantages encountered with the traditional methods used for genetic material delivery. The application of nanoparticles in gene delivery is illustrated in Chapter 2. Compared to polymeric nanoparticles, lipid-based nanoparticles have long been perceived as the more ideal drug delivery vehicles because of their superior biocompatibility. In Chapter 3, lipid-based nano drug delivery systems that are currently being investigated are discussed along with optimization and in vitro characterization procedures. To address the limitations of polymeric nanoparticles and lipid nanocarriers, a new generation delivery vehicle of therapeutics, termed hybrid nanoparticles, has drawn the attention of researchers. Therefore, the drug delivery applications of hybrid nanocarriers have been included in Chapter 4. This is followed by Chapter 5 that discloses the potential of mucosal route for improving olfactory drug delivery. Chapter 6 illustrates plasma drug delivery in order to enhance percutaneous absorption of drugs, an approach different from the use of conventional skin permeation enhancers. Till now, the safe and efficient delivery of therapeutic genes to the diseased cells has been a major challenge. Although viral vectors display good transduction properties, the safety issues are still to be solved. Meanwhile, considerable progress has been noticed in developing biopolymer-based non-viral expression vectors. Hence, Chapter 7 has been devoted to a discussion on potential application of biomaterial as non-viral vectors for gene delivery. The assistance of nuclear medicine in identifying drug delivery system in the body and its biodistribution characteristics is deeply appreciated in Chapter 8.

Hopefully, these topics will enrich readers with better understanding, broad perspectives, and an insight into the current state and future promises. This book would serve as a useful resource for pharmacy students, teaching professionals, medical and biomedical researchers, and those working in the field of polymer and biological sciences.

The book is aimed at those who are interested in understanding the fundamentals and progress of drug delivery technology. We would be happy if the content of this book creates interest among pharmaceutical scientists and augment the drug delivery research in bringing novel formulations for the benefit of humanity.

We would like to express our sincere gratitude to all the authors for their contribution to accomplish this book project. The various sources of information related to the content of our book are cited in each chapter and are gratefully acknowledged. We are also thankful to our family members who motivated us for the successful completion of this book project. We are thankful to InTech publisher for their keen interest and expert assistance in the publication of the book.

Dr. Sabyasachi Maiti
Professor,
Department of Pharmaceutics,
Gupta College of Technological Sciences, Asansol,
West Bengal, India

Dr. Kalyan Kumar Sen
Principal & Professor,
Department of Pharmaceutics,
Gupta College of Technological Sciences,
Asansol, West Bengal, India

Chapter 1

Introductory Chapter: Drug Delivery Concepts

Sabyasachi Maiti and Kalyan Kumar Sen

Additional information is available at the end of the chapter

http://dx.doi.org/10.5772/65245

1. Introduction

Drug delivery systems (DDSs) are pharmaceutical formulations or devices that help in achieving targeted delivery and/or controlled release (CR) of therapeutic agents in our body [1]. Following administration, the DDSs liberate the active ingredients, and subsequently, the bioactive molecules are transported across various biological barriers to reach the site of action. The scientists have contributed substantially to understand the role of different physiological barriers in efficient transport of drugs in the circulatory system and drug movement through cells and tissues. In addition, their significant contribution to the development of a number of new modes of drug delivery has entered clinical practice. Despite a significant advancement in the process of new drug design and discovery, many drugs have unacceptable side effects due to interaction of the drug with parts of the body that are not the target for the drug. Sometimes, side effects occur depending on the medication, the mode of delivery, and response from our body. The buildup of high blood plasma drug concentration due to accumulation of drug from repeated administration of conventional DDS may lead to untoward side effects. Hence, the attempts must be made to afford better patient compliance effect from the reduction in the number and frequency of doses needed to maintain the desired therapeutic responses. These side effects can vary greatly from person to person in type and severity. The method by which the drug is delivered can have a significant impact on its efficacy.

It is necessary to develop suitable DDS for all drugs to allow their effective and safe application to the patient. Indeed, DDSs control the drug release rate and drug absorption and ultimately the therapeutic effects along with side effects of the drug. Ideal DDSs ensure that the active drug is available at the site of action according to the need of patient for an intended duration. The drug concentration at the appropriate site should remain in the therapeutic

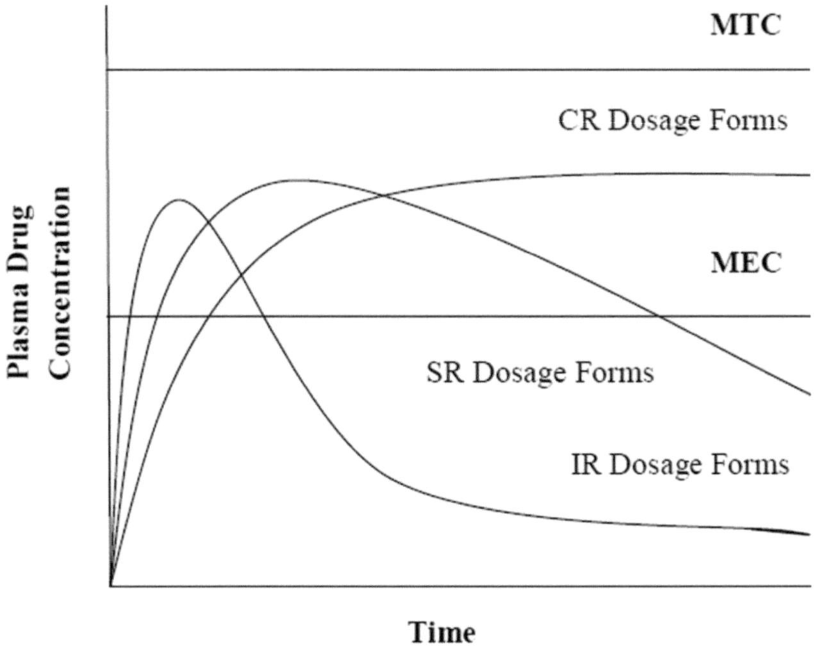

Figure 1. The drug plasma levels after single oral administration of a drug from (a) IR dosage form, (b) SR dosage form, and (c) CR dosage form.

window, that is, between minimal effective concentration (MEC) and minimal toxic concentration (MTC). This concept is illustrated in **Figure 1**.

The maintenance of drug concentration in therapeutic range depends on the frequency of dosing, the drug clearance rates, the route of administration, and the DDS employed. Some drugs have an optimum concentration range within which maximum benefit is derived, and concentrations above or below this range can be toxic or produce no therapeutic benefit at all. DDS can be classified according to their physical state, site/route of administration, and the rate of drug release. The dosage form may be gaseous (e.g., anesthetics), liquid (e.g., solutions, emulsions, and suspensions), semisolid (e.g., creams, ointments, and gels), and solid dosage (e.g., tablets and capsules) [2]. Drugs can be administered directly into the body through injection or infusion termed parenteral drug delivery. Depending on the site of administration, one can differentiate among intravenous, intramuscular, subcutaneous, intradermal, and intraperitoneal administration. Mostly semisolid dosage forms including creams, ointments, and gels are applied onto the skin to enter into the body. However, the liquid dosage forms, such as emulsions, or solid dosage forms, such as transdermal patches, can also be used. Dosage forms can be classified into immediate release (IR) and modified release (MR). IR dosage forms allow the drug to dissolve in the gastrointestinal contents, without delaying or prolonging the dissolution or absorption of the drug. In MR dosage forms, the time course and/or location of drug release is chosen to accomplish therapeutic or convenience objectives not offered by conventional dosage forms. MR dosage forms include both delayed and extended release drug products.

Delayed release dosage forms release the active ingredient at a time other than immediately after administration, for example, enteric-coated dosage forms or colon-specific dosage forms. These systems delay the release of drug until the dosage form reaches the small intestine. In this way, they can protect the drug from degradation in the low-pH environment of the stomach or protect the stomach from irritation by the drug. The dosage form is coated with polymer that dissolves and releases the drug at higher pH during its travel from low-pH environment of the stomach to the high-pH environment of the small intestine. Once this occurs, the release is again immediate, and the resulting plasma concentration versus time curve is similar to the one for IR dosage forms. Extended release products (sustained release (SR) and controlled release systems) are formulated to make the drug available over an extended period after ingestion. This allows a reduction in dosing frequency compared to the drug presented as a conventional dosage form. IR dosage forms are designed to achieve quicker onset of drug action than that achieved by delayed or extended release dosage forms, which are often desirable to increase the stability, safety, and efficacy of the drug, to improve the therapeutic outcome of the drug treatment, and/or to increase patient compliance and convenience of administration.

The extended release DDS can be of either sustained release (SR) or controlled release (CR) dosage forms. The polymer-based matrix or reservoir sustained release systems maintain the rate of drug release over a longer period and reduce the frequency of dosing. Conversely, CR DDSs are designed to predict constant plasma drug concentrations regardless of the biological environment of the application site. Therefore, CR systems actually control the drug concentration in the body, whereas SR systems just regulate the release of the drug from the dosage form [3, 4]. Further, SR systems are basically restricted to oral formulations, while CR systems can be administered through various routes, including transdermal, oral, and vaginal administration.

Ideally, the release rate from the dosage form should be the rate-determining step for drug absorption and in fact for the drug concentration in the plasma and target site. The resulting plasma concentration versus time curves become increasingly flatter from IR to extended release dosage forms, indicating the prolonged maintenance of drug in the therapeutic range after a single administration of the dosage form. Controlled DDSs have been introduced to overwhelm the drawback of fluctuating drug levels associated with conventional dosage forms [5]. Controlled drug release and subsequent biodegradation are important for developing successful formulations. The release mechanisms involve desorption of surface-bound/adsorbed drugs; diffusion through the carrier matrix or polymer membrane surrounding drug core; matrix erosion; combination of erosion/diffusion process; and responsiveness to stimuli such as light, changes in pH, or temperature.

The formulation scientist must optimize the bioavailability of the drug. To achieve this goal, the delivery systems should allow the drug to reach the systemic circulation, more importantly to the target site in the body to avoid side effects by preventing the exposure of drug to the nontarget sites. In addition, the drug must be physically and chemically compatible with the formulation excipients in the dosage forms and stable microbiologically. The delivery systems should be designed in such a way that it can improve the patient compliance. One can design an oral dosage form instead of parenteral formulations for the drug, which can allow self-administration of the dosage forms. Moreover, the pharmaceutical quality of the delivery systems must be ensured in accordance with the regulatory specifications to facilitate reproducible drug release from the system and minimize the influence of the body such as food effects on drug release. It is also necessary to investigate the feasibility of the developed DDS to be scaled up from the laboratory to the production scale.

However, controlled release systems do not exclusively deliver the drug to the target organ. For this reason, the target-specific drug delivery systems must be designed in order to control biodistribution of the drug. Consequently, various novel concepts have been emerged to meet the specific needs of an ideal drug delivery system. This chapter introduces a brief description of targeted drug delivery mechanism along with some of the novel-targeted drug delivery options.

2. Targeted drug delivery

Very few drugs bind selectively to the desired therapeutic target, and hence, some targeting approaches are required to destine the drug in desired tissue or organ to reduce efficacy and dose-related toxicity. The concept of targeted drugs is not new, but dates back to 1960 when Paul Ehrlich first postulated the concept of "magic bullet," and this continues to be a challenge to implement in the clinic. The challenges include the selection of proper target for a particular disease, drug for effective treatment and stable, biodegradable drug carriers while avoiding the immunogenic and nonspecific interactions that efficiently clear foreign material from the body. Moreover, the preparation of the delivery system should be easy or reasonably simple, reproductive, and cost-effective. Nanoparticles (NPs) are potentially useful as carriers of active drugs and, when coupled with targeting ligands, may fulfill many attributes of a "magic bullet." Furthermore, the NPs offer several potential advantages including increased efficacy and therapeutic index, improved pharmacokinetic effect, reproducible sizes with opportunity for surface functionalization, ability to entrap both hydrophilic and lipophilic drug, increasing stability of drug from enzymatic degradation, thereby delivering entrapped drug intact to various tissue and cells for site-specific and targeted delivery and thus decreasing drug toxicity. The size and other characteristics can be manipulated depending on the drug and intended use of the product [6]. The drug targeting strategies must meet two basic requirements to achieve effective drug delivery. The drugs should reach the desired sites after administration, with minimal loss of the dose and activity in blood circulation. Second, the drugs should act only on target cells without harmful effects to healthy tissue [7]. Two strategies have been adopted for drug targeting: *passive targeting* and *active targeting*.

2.1. Passive targeting

Passive targeting exploits natural conditions of the target organ or tissue to direct the drug to the target site. For example, passive targeting takes advantage of the unique pathophysiological characteristics of tumor vessels, that is, leaky vasculature with 100–800 nm pores enabling nanodrugs to accumulate in tumor tissues. Typically, tumor vessels are highly disorganized and dilated with a high number of pores, resulting in enlarged gap junctions between endothelial cells and compromised lymphatic drainage. The leaky vascularization, coupled with poor lymphatic drainage, serves to enhance the permeation and retention of NPs within the tumor region. This is often called enhanced permeability and retention (EPR) effect [8]. The drug-loaded NPs are preferentially accumulated in tumor tissue than normal cells, solely due to their small particle size rather than binding. The NPs cannot readily cross the blood capillaries of normal tissues because they are held up with tight junctions. Therefore, passive targeting approach can assist in depositing a higher amount of drug in solid tumors than that of free drug.

In addition to the EPR effect, the passive targeting is supported by microenvironment surrounding tumor tissue that is different from that of healthy cells. The fast-growing tumor cells require more oxygen and nutrients to maintain high metabolic rate. Consequently, glycolysis is stimulated to acquire more energy and creates an acidic environment [9]. This advantage can be exploited to target chemotherapeutic agents to the tumor cells. The pH-sensitive NPs have been prepared that remain stable at physiological pH 7.4 but degrade at the acidic pH of the tumor and liberate the drug molecules. In case of cancer treatment, the size and surface properties of drug delivery NPs must be controlled specifically to avoid uptake by the reticuloendothelial system (RES) to maximize circulation times and targeting ability [10].

2.2. Active targeting

One way to overcome the limitations of passive targeting is to attach ligands such as antibodies, peptides, vitamins, aptamers, or small molecules by a variety of conjugation chemistries to the surface of the nanocarriers that only bind to specific receptors on the cell surface [11]. For high specificity, however, the receptors need to be highly expressed on tumor cells rather than on normal cells. The targeting conjugates are internalized by receptor-mediated endocytosis mechanism. The targeting ligands bind with the receptors first, followed by endosome formation with the enclosure of the ligand-receptor complex by plasma membrane. The endosome is then transferred to specific organelles, and drugs are released by acidic pH or enzymes.

3. Novel delivery modalities

To prevent chemical degradation, harmful side effects, and improve drug bioavailability and accumulation in the desired site, various drug delivery and drug targeting systems are currently under development. The delivery carriers can be made slowly degradable, stimuli-responsive (e.g., pH, ionic strength, temperature, ultrasound, light, electricity, enzymes), and even targeted (e.g., by conjugating them with specific ligands). Over last two decades, nanotechnology has shown potential benefits in improving drug delivery and targeting properties and therefore opens up new markets for pharmaceutical and drug delivery companies. The drug delivery systems are also designed to overcome some physical barriers, such as the blood-brain barrier (BBB) for better location and effectiveness of the drug at the target site. Due to their small size, the NPs can pass through certain biological barriers.

Polymeric NPs are colloidal particles with a size range of 10–1000 nm, which are fabricated using biodegradable synthetic polymers, such as poly (lactide-*co*-glycolide), polyacrylates, and polycaprolactones; nonbiodegradable synthetic polymers, such as poly (methyl methacrylate), polyacrylamide, poly (vinyl alcohol), and poly (ethylene glycol); or natural polymers, such as albumin, gelatin, alginate, gellan gum, and chitosan [12]. Sometimes, blends or graft copolymers of natural and synthetic polymers are also used. In recent years, biodegradable polymeric NPs have attracted considerable attention in the fabrication of potential drug delivery devices due to easy removal of degraded fragments from the body via normal metabolic pathways.

Various methods, such as solvent evaporation, spontaneous emulsification, solvent diffusion, salting out/emulsification-diffusion, and polymerization, have been used to prepare the NPs [13]. Depending upon the method of preparation of NPs, the drug is confined to a cavity surrounded by a polymer membrane (nanocapsules) or dispersed physically and uniformly in the polymer matrix (nanospheres). The drug is loaded via hydrophobic interactions between drugs and nanocarriers. The drug can also be conjugated to polymeric carriers via covalent chemistry.

An important feature of targeted particle delivery system is the ability to simultaneously carry a high amount of drug while displaying ligands on the surface of particles. The overall binding strength of NPs to target is a function of both the affinity of the ligand-target interaction and the number of targeting ligands present on the particle surface [14].

The drug-loaded particles are internalized into cells in determining their biological activity. The particles of as large as 500 nm size can be internalized by nonphagocytic cells via energy-dependent process. The particles with <200 nm diameter are internalized via clathrin-coated pits, but larger ones are taken up by cells via caveolae membrane invaginations [15]. However, the internalization of particles can be mediated independent of both clathrin and caveolae pathways. To facilitate efficient internalization, NPs have been targeted against internalizing receptors, and an increased therapeutic activity has been observed in some tumor models [16, 17].

Targeting ligands include any molecule that recognizes and binds to target antigen or receptors overexpressed or selectively expressed by particular cells or tissue components. The antibodies or their fragments, peptides, glycoproteins, vitamins, or carbohydrates are the common class of ligands. The NPs are made long circulating by making their surface hydrophilic after coupling or coating poly(ethylene glycol) (PEG). Functionality could also be introduced by incorporating PEG with functional end groups for coupling to target ligands.

There has been a considerable progress in the field of gene delivery using polymeric NPs. For gene delivery, the plasmid DNA is introduced into the target cells, and the genetic information is ultimately translated into the corresponding protein [18]. To achieve this, an efficient vector that possesses high transfection efficiency, biodegradability, targeting ability, DNA protecting ability, stimuli sensitivity, and low cytotoxicity for delivering a target gene to specific tissues or cells must be selected to cure both the genetic and acquired diseases of human [19]. Despite more gene transfection efficiency, viral vectors may pose a significant risk to patients, while nonviral carriers are inherently safer than viral carriers [20]. Furthermore, the nonviral carriers are expected to be less immunogenic with a possible versatile surface modification [21]. The nonviral vectors are usually made of lipids or polymers with/without using other inorganic materials. The NPs can protect genes against nuclease degradation and improve their stability [22]. Furthermore, they can be used for targeted delivery purpose. Because the biopolymers are non-toxic, biodegradable, and biocompatible, the biopolymer-based non-viral vectors are also being tested for safe and efficient gene delivery.

The liposomes are the most clinically established nanosystems for drug delivery. They are self-assembled spherical vesicles of bilayer structures of phospholipids and cholesterol surrounding an aqueous core, and their size can be controlled as small as 50–100 nm. The vesicles are biocompatible and biodegradable and confer the ability to entrap both hydrophilic and hydrophobic drugs. The variation in composition of lipid membrane and surface chemistry, the liposome properties, such as size, surface charge, and functionality can be easily manipulated. The incorporation of polyethylene glycol (PEG) prevents interactions with plasma proteins, retards recognition by the RES [23], and thus enhances the liposome circulation lifetime, that is, stealth liposomes. Liposomes can also be conjugated with active-targeting ligands, such as antibodies or folate for target-specific drug delivery. Their efficacy has been demonstrated in reducing systemic effects and toxicity, as well as in attenuating drug clearance [24]. Despite potential advantages, the liposomes as targeted drug delivery carriers are associated with some major drawbacks like poor control over drug release rate, leakage of drug into the blood, low encapsulation efficiency, industrial scale-up, and poor storage stability [25, 26].

Recently, extensive work and experiments with solid lipids resulted in the invention of lipid-based solid particles in the submicron range (10–1000 nm). These NPs are made up of biocompatible and biodegradable lipids with potential application in drug delivery. They possess a solid lipid core matrix that can solubilize lipophilic molecules for enhancing bioavailability. The physiologically similar lipid core of triglycerides or fatty acids or waxes is stabilized by surfactants (emulsifiers). All classes of emulsifiers (with respect to charge and molecular weight) can be used to stabilize the lipid dispersion. It has been found that an emulsifier combination may prevent particle agglomeration more efficiently [27]. The lipid NPs combine the advantages of lipid emulsion and polymeric NPs while overcoming the temporal and *in vivo* stability issues that trouble the conventional and nanoscale delivery approaches [28]. A variety of materials can be used to engineer solid NPs for targeting tissues by either passive or active targeting.

Lipid-polymer hybrid NPs are core-shell structures comprising polymer cores and lipid shells, which exhibit complementary characteristics of both polymeric NPs and liposomes, particularly in terms of their physical stability, biocompatibility, and *in vivo* cellular delivery efficacy [29]. In core-shell-type lipid-polymer hybrid NPs, a biodegradable polymeric core is surrounded by a shell composed of phospholipid layers. The hybrid architecture can provide advantages such as controllable particle size, surface functionality, high loading of multiple drugs, tunable drug release profile, and good serum stability [30].

Several drugs do not have adequate physiochemical characteristics such as high lipid solubility, low molecular size, and positive charge, to traverse blood-brain barrier and deliver drug into the brain [31]. Therefore, the delivery of drugs to central nervous system (CNS) is a challenge for treating neurological disorders. The drugs may be administered directly into the CNS or administered systematically for targeted action in the CNS. The osmotic and chemical opening of the blood-brain barrier as well as the transport/carrier systems constitutes some of the widely reported strategies to promote the permeation of blood-brain barrier (BBB) and delivery of drugs in brain. In conjunction with the net delivery of drug, the access to the intended target site within the CNS is also important. To serve this purpose, the drugs may be conjugated with various nanostructures such as liposomes and NPs and a suitable route of administration can be sought. It has been postulated that nanoscale drug carriers possess a great potential for improving the delivery of drugs through nasal routes to deliver drugs to the brain. Among other mucosal sites, nasal delivery is especially attractive for brain-targeted drug delivery, as the nasal epithelium is characterized by its relatively high permeability, vuscularized mucosa, and low enzymatic activity. If a nasal drug formulation is delivered deep and high enough into the nasal cavity, the olfactory mucosa may be reached and drug transport into the brain and/or cerebrospinal fluid (CSF) via the olfactory receptor neurons may occur [32].

Transdermal systems in the form of patches deliver the drugs across the skin barrier for systemic effects at a predetermined and controlled rate. Due to concentration gradient between the transdermal patch and blood, the drug will continue diffusing into the blood for prolonged period of time and maintain constant drug concentration in the blood flow. Transdermal drug delivery avoids problems such as gastrointestinal irritation, metabolism, pH-dependent variation in delivery rate, and interference with gastric emptying due to presence of food. However, slow penetration rates, lack of dosage flexibility and/or precision, and a restriction to relatively low dosage drugs are the major limitations. The stratum corneum of the skin forms a formidable barrier against uptake, and thus transdermal delivery is difficult to achieve. The substances having molecular weight greater than 500 Da [33] and hydrophilic characteristics encounter the difficulty in absorption through skin. Penetration enhancers often have to be added to the delivery system to improve delivery into or through the skin. Recently, it has been demonstrated that atmospheric-pressure argon microplasma irradiation (AAMI) can improve skin permeability of drugs without the need of injection needles and skin damages [34]. AAMI can be a promising alternative to promote drug delivery through the skin and simultaneously minimize the pain from other manipulations related to skin penetration enhancement. However, the feasibility of atmospheric microplasma irradiation is still under investigation for enhancing percutaneous absorption of drugs.

The delivery of drug to a specific target in the body is comparable to the magic bullet principle applied in nuclear medicine. Nuclear medicine may advance drug development by visualizing biodistribution and site of action [35]. The biodistribution and release kinetics of drug from the novel formulations can be quantified by radiolabeling with γ-emitting radionuclide. Many nuclear medicine departments have participated in the assessment of drug performance and toxicity in contributing data to clinical trials. The application of nuclear medicine techniques to the evaluation of pharmaceutical formulations has been an interesting area of work. Scintigraphy can be used to determine the position of drug release and assess site-specific absorption of orally administered drugs, for example, the evaluation of controlled release formulation designed to release the drug specifically in colon [36]. Hence, the importance of nuclear medicine in drug delivery application has been described in detail in this book.

http://dx.doi.org/10.5772/65245

4. Future considerations

The new delivery methods could enhance the performance of drugs by increasing effectiveness, safety, and patient compliance and ultimately reduce healthcare costs. Nanotechnology could be strategically implemented in developing new drug delivery systems that can expand drug markets. Nanomaterials are poised to take advantage of existing cellular machinery to facilitate the delivery of drugs. However, clinical development of drugs is halted because of poor biopharmaceutical and undesirable pharmacokinetic properties. Novel delivery technologies are being tested for overcoming the barriers toward safe delivery of drugs. An in-depth understanding of novel strategies constitutes the primary focus and subsequent demonstration of easy scale-up of the formulations with favorable pharmacokinetics and toxicity profiles could augment the translation of research findings into practical therapeutics. A collaborative effort among scientists in various disciplines, including medicine, materials science, engineering, physics, and biotechnology could potentiate the translation of novel laboratory innovation into commercially viable medical products.

Author details

Sabyasachi Maiti* and Kalyan Kumar Sen

*Address all correspondence to: sabya245@rediffmail.com

Department of Pharmaceutics, Gupta College of Technological Sciences, Asansol, West Bengal, India

References

[1] Jain KK. Drug delivery systems – an overview. Methods Mol. Biol. 2008; **437**:1–50. doi:10.1007/978-1-59745-210-6_1.

[2] Perrie Y, Rades T. FASTtrack Pharmaceutics: Drug Delivery and Targeting. 2nd ed. London: Pharmaceutical Press; 2012. p. 1–24.

[3] Ballard BE. An overview of prolonged action drug dosage forms. In: Robinson JR, editor. Sustained and Controlled Release Drug Delivery Systems. 1st ed. New York: Marcel Dekker, Inc.; 1978. p. 3–8.

[4] Chien YW. 1992. Novel drug delivery systems. In: Swarbrick J, editor. Drugs and the Pharmaceutical Sciences. 2nd ed. New York: Marcel Dekker, Inc.; 1992. p. 1–2.

[5] Vyas SP, Khar RK. Controlled Drug Delivery: Concepts and Advances. 1st ed. New Delhi: Vallabh Prakashan; 2006. p. 1–53.

[6] Vyas SP, Khar RK. Targeted and Controlled Drug Delivery. 1st ed. New Delhi: CBS Publishers and Distributors; 2008. p. 42–46.

[7] Cho K, Wang X, Nie S, Chen Z, Shin DM. Therapeutic nanoparticles for drug delivery in cancer. Clin. Cancer Res. 2008; **14**:1310–1316. doi:10.1158/1078-0432.CCR-07-1441.

[8] Sledge GW Jr, Miller KD. Exploiting the hallmarks of cancer: the future conquest of breast cancer. Eur. J. Cancer. 2003; **39**:1668–1675. doi:10.1016/S0959-8049(03)00273-9.

[9] Pelicano H, Martin DS, Xu RH, Huang P. Glycolysis inhibition for anticancer treatment. Oncogene. 2006; **25**:4633–4646. doi:10.1038/sj.onc.1209597.

[10] Gref R, Minamitake Y, Peracchia MT, Trubetskoy V, Torchilin V, Langer R. Biodegradable long-circulating polymeric nanospheres. Science. 1994; **263**:1600–1603. doi:10.1126/science.8128245.

[11] Bamrungsap S, Zhao Z, Chen T, Wang L, Li C, Fu T, Tan W. Nanotechnology in therapeutics – a focus on nanoparticles as a drug delivery system. Nanomedicine. 2012; **7**:1253–1271. doi:10.2217/nnm.12.87.

[12] Panyam J, Labhasetwar V. Biodegradable nanoparticles for drug and gene delivery to cells and tissue. Adv. Drug Deliv. Rev. 2003; **55**:329–347. doi:10.1016/S0169-409X(02)00228-4.

[13] Soppimath KS, Aminabhavi TM, Kulkarni AR, Rudzinski WE. Biodegradable polymeric nanoparticles as drug delivery devices. J. Control. Release. 2001; **70**:1–20. doi:10.1016/S0168-3659(00)00339-4.

[14] Adams GP, Schier R, Marshall K, Wolf EJ, McCall AM, Marks JD, Weiner LM. Increased affinity leads to improved selective tumor delivery of single-chain Fv antibodies. Cancer Res. 1998; **58**:485–490. PMID: 9458094.

[15] Koval M, Preiter K, Adles C, Stahl PD, Steinberg TH. Size of IgG-opsonized particles determines macrophage response during internalization. Exp. Cell Res. 1998; **242**:265–273. doi:10.1006/excr.1998.4110.

[16] Sugano M, Egilmez NK, Yokota SJ, Chen FA, Harding J, Huang SK, Bankert RB. Antibody targeting of doxorubicin-loaded liposomes suppresses the growth and metastatic spread of established human lung tumor xenografts in severe combined immunodeficient mice. Cancer Res. 2000; **60**:6942–6949. PubMed 11156394.

[17] Park JW, Hong K, Kirpotin DB, Colbern G, Shalaby R, Baselga J, Shao Y, Nielsen UB, Marks JD, Moore D, Papahadjopoulos D, Benz CC. Anti-HER2 immunoliposomes: enhanced efficacy attributable to targeted delivery. Clin. Cancer Res. 2002; **8**:1172–1181. PubMed 11948130.

[18] Tian H, Chen J, Chen X. Nanoparticles for gene delivery. Small. 2013; **9**:2034–2044. doi:10.1002/smll.201202485.

[19] Dizaj SM, Jafari S, Khosroushahi AY. A sight on the current nanoparticle-based gene delivery vectors. Nanoscale Res. Lett. 2014; **9**:252–260. doi:10.1186/1556-276X-9-252.

[20] Mastrobattista E, van der Aa MA, Hennink WE, Crommelin DJ. Artificial viruses: a nanotechnological approach to gene delivery. Nat. Rev. Drug Discov. 2006; **5**:115–121. doi:10.1038/nrd1960.

[21] Philippi C, Loretz B, Schaefer UF, Lehr CM. Telomerase as an emerging target to fight cancer-opportunities and challenges for nanomedicine. J. Control. Release. 2010; **146**:228–240. doi:10.1016/j.jconrel.2010.03.025.

[22] Morachis JM, Mahmoud EA, Sankaranarayanan J, Almutairi A. Triggered rapid degradation of nanoparticles for gene delivery. J. Drug Deliv. 2012; **2012**:1–7. doi:10.1155/2012/291219.

[23] Gabizon A, Shmeeda H, Barenholz Y. Pharmacokinetics of pegylated liposomal doxorubicin: review of animal and human studies. Clin. Pharmacokinet. 2003; **42**:419–436. doi:10.2165/00003088-200342050-00002.

[24] Torchilin VP. Recent advances with liposomes as pharmaceutical carriers. Nat. Rev. Drug Discov. 2005; **4**:145–160. doi:10.1038/nrd1632.

[25] Soppimath KS, Aminabhavi TM, Kulkarni AR, Rudzinski WE. Biodegradable polymeric nanoparticles as drug delivery devices. J. Control. Release. 2001; **70**:1–20. doi:10.1016/S0168-3659(00)00339-4.

[26] Hans ML, Lowman AM. Biodegradable nanoparticles for drug delivery and targeting. Curr. Opin. Solid State Mater. Sci. 2002; **6**:319–327. doi:10.1016/S1359-0286(02)00117-1.

[27] Mashaghi S, Jadidi T, Koenderink G, Mashaghi A. Lipid nanotechnology. Int. J. Mol. Sci. 2013; **14**:4242–4282. doi:10.3390/ijms14024242.

[28] Mehnert W, Mäder K. Solid lipid nanoparticles: production, characterization and applications. Adv. Drug Deliv. Rev. 2001; **47**:165–196. doi:10.1016/S0169-409X(01)00105-3.

[29] Hadinoto K, Sundaresan A, Cheow WS. Lipid-polymer hybrid nanoparticles as a new generation therapeutic delivery platform: a review. Eur. J. Pharm. Biopharm. 2013; **85**:427–443. doi:10.1016/j.ejpb.2013.07.002.

[30] Mandal B, Bhattacharjee H, Mittal N, Sah H, Balabathula P, Thoma LA, Wood GC. Core-shell-type lipid-polymer hybrid nanoparticles as a drug delivery platform. Nanomedicine. 2013; **9**:474–491. doi:10.1016/j.nano.2012.11.010.

[31] Banerjee G, Nandi G, Mahato SB, Pakrashi A, Basu MK. Drug delivery system: targeting of pentamidines to specific sites using sugar grafted liposomes. J. Antimicrob. Chemother. 1996; **38**:145–150. doi:10.1093/jac/38.1.145.

[32] Sharma D, Chelvi TP, Kaur J, Chakravorty K, De TK, Maitra A, Ralhan R. Novel taxol formulation: polyvinylpyrrolidone nanoparticles encapsulated taxol for drug delivery in cancer therapy. Oncol. Res. 1996; **8**:281–286. PMID: 8938791.

[33] Prausnitz MR, Langer R. Transdermal drug delivery. Nat. Biotechnol. 2008; **26**:1261–1268. doi:10.1038/nbt.1504.

[34] Shimizu K, Hayashida K, Blajan M. Novel method to improve transdermal drug delivery by atmospheric microplasma irradiation. Biointerphases 2015; **10**:029517. doi:10.1116/1.4919708.

[35] Leitha T. Nuclear medicine: proof of principle for targeted drugs in diagnosis and therapy. Curr. Pharm. Des. 2009; **15**:173–187.

[36] Perkins A, Frier M. Nuclear medicine imaging and drug delivery. Nucl. Med. Commun. 2000; **21**:415–416. PMID: 10874696.

Chapter 2

Medicated Nanoparticle for Gene Delivery

Sakthivel Lakshmana Prabu ,
Timmadonu Narasimman Kuppusami Suriyaprakash and
Rathinasabapathy Thirumurugan

Additional information is available at the end of the chapter

http://dx.doi.org/10.5772/65709

Abstract

Delivering the drug to the target site with a desired concentration to provide therapeutic effect is a major problem in the drug delivery system. Effectiveness, poor distribution and lack of selectivity are the drawbacks of the conventional dosage form. Recently Nanotechnology has been given much attention in various fields specifically in the biomedical application. Material includes organic, inorganic, polymeric and lipid-based nanobiomaterials after surface modification; it has been utilized for drug and gene delivery systems. Viral and non-viral vectors are the two types in gene delivery utilizing genetic materials like DNA plasmids, RNA and siRNA. Cellular and extracellular barriers are the two main barriers in gene delivery. The basic mechanism involved in the gene delivery is an introduction of a gene encoding a functional protein altering the expression of an endogenous gene or owning the capacity to cure or prevent the progression of a disease. Nanoparticle surface features like particle shape and surface charge are having major roles in the gene delivery. To provide the site-specific delivery various properties like nature of polymer, particle size, solubility, biocompatibility, biodegradability and nanoparticle surface features are need to be considered. Gene delivery has been utilized for various disease treatments such as cancer, AIDS, and cardiovascular diseases.

Keywords: Gene delivery, DNA, RNA, Nanoparticle

1. Introduction

Drug and gene delivery system include organic, inorganic, polymeric and lipid-based nanobiomaterials. Binding of the nanobiomaterials to the receptors to target cells/tissues can be improved by surface modification. This surface modification may increase solubility, immune compatibility, and cellular uptake.

Various nano drug delivery systems include nanoparticles, nanocapsules, nanotubes, nanogels, and dendrimers. They can be used to deliver both small molecule drugs and various classes of biomacromolecules, such as peptides, proteins, plasmid DNA, and synthetic oligodeoxynucleotides. Antisense oligonucleotide (AS-ODN) and small interfering RNA (siRNA) are shown as promise one in gene delivery and good therapeutic agents, but it can be used directly due to their limitations such as sequence size, length, charge, half-life, or stability in solutions [1].

Various diseases are occurred in human beings due to mutations or deletions in genes lead to metabolic pathway disorder, regulation of cell cycle, protein function and its structure, function of receptor, and cell skeleton [2]. This can be treated effectively through gene delivery system. Gene delivery is a term used when referring to the delivery of genetic material such as DNA plasmids, RNA, and siRNA into target cells either encapsulated inside or conjugated to the NPs to express or suppress the biosynthesis of proteins (also called transfection) to treat or cure many diseases [3–10].

2. Various gene delivery mechanisms

2.1. Plasmid DNA

It is currently the most commonly investigated nucleic acid in gene delivery applications. When the pDNA is entering into the nucleus, the pDNA strand is transcribed, and the coding gene is translated to protein, which is then expressed from the cell.

2.2. RNA interference

It is triggered by double-stranded RNA (dsRNA), activates the anti-viral interferon leads to shutdown of protein synthesis by degradation of messenger RNA (mRNA). Another mechanism involves the use of microRNAs (miRNA), which are small non-coding nucleic acids responsible for post-translational regulation of protein expression.

2.3. Small interfering RNA

Small interfering RNA comprises around 21–23 nucleotides, which can be designed to be better targeted than long dsRNA and can eliminate the activation of the response of the interferon while still inhibiting target gene expression. The gene expression can be able to control/block transected siRNA into mammalian cells; this specific gene block can be used to treat certain infectious diseases and cancers [11–14].

To obtain an efficient vector system and to achieve a high rate of cell transfection, the following two limitations must be integrated in the development of an ideal genetic vector. In the gene transfer methods whether viral, physical, or chemical, these two major limitations must be overcome.

1. The first limitation is a carrier, which is needed to carry the nucleic acids to the target cells without potential risks. Naturally viruses having the ability to recognize and locate the defined target cells due to its body defense mechanisms, such as the reticulo-endothelial system (RES). Whereas the chemical vectors conjugate with targeting molecules to realize the specific location through various techniques.

2. The second limitation is the penetration of the nucleic acids into the cell through the plasma membrane. Viruses can achieve the same through natural mechanisms, whereas the chemical vectors must disturb the plasma membrane (e.g. physical vectors)/or internal vesicular membranes (e.g. the cationic lipids) [15].

3. Gene delivery

In gene delivery, a vector/carrier is essential in order to carry the hydrophilic, negatively charged DNA through the hydrophobic and negatively charged cell membrane. The therapeutic efficiency depends upon the efficient delivery of DNA into the target site. Barriers including cellular like intracellular uptake, endosomal escape, DNA release, and nuclear uptake and extracellular barriers like avoidance of particle clearance mechanisms, targeting to specific tissues and/or cells of interest, and protection of DNA from degradation are present in the system [16–19]. One main hurdle in gene delivery is the delivery of therapeutic polynucleotides crossing the plasma membrane and delivering into the cells of interest. This is the limitation one in the gene delivery for efficient and safe delivery into the cells. A good gene delivery vector should be able to effectively compact and protect DNA, sufficient stability during bypassing the immune system of the host, traverse the plasma membrane (typically through endocytosis), disrupt the endosomal membrane, and deliver the DNA into the nucleus [20–22]. Successful gene transfer requires sufficient stability of DNA during the extracellular delivery phase, transportation through cell membranes, cytoplasm, and eventual disassembly and nuclear delivery.

Gene delivery systems can be divided into two general categories:

1. Viral transduction systems

2. Nonviral transfection systems

Initially, viruses were used for gene delivery. The disadvantages of viral vectors limited their application in gene delivery like due to its size of DNA that they can carry, low loading capacity, large-scale manufacturing, quality control cost, and safety factor such as immunogenicity and potential oncogenicity [23].

Hence, more attention has been paid to develop non-viral vectors as an alternative one for gene delivery [6, 8–10, 24].

Nonviral delivery systems have advantages like easy to prepare, amenable to synthetic manipulations of polymer properties, cell/tissue targeting, less immunogenic and oncogenic, no potential of virus recombination and limitation on the size of a transferred gene, virtually no limitation on the unrestricted plasmid size that can be delivered and the cost of production is relatively low [25]. Moreover, they can be consigned readily to carry genetic materials to target cells by virtue of their size, charge and structurally modifying the vectors [26]. Difference between viral and nonviral gene delivery is based on the various gene transfer and its complementary mechanisms. The mechanism includes in the viral gene delivery is the ability of virus to circulate in the blood, bind to cell surface receptors, gain entry into the cell, avoid lysosomal destruction, survive degradation in the cytosol, and deliver genetic material to the nucleus. In the nonviral gene delivery overcoming biological barriers in the circulation or inside the target cell and transferring the gene vector is based on the molecular weight of the vector, ratio between the vector nitrogens and the DNA phosphates (termed the N:P ratio) and the salt concentration of the buffer solution. [27–30].

Nonviral gene delivery systems are typically composed of plasmid DNA condensed into nanoparticles by a cationic polymer [31].

Nonviral vectors are categories into lipid- and polymer-based one. Whereas the polymeric based nonviral vectors have the advantage over lipid-based one due to its modification property.

The steps involved in the polymeric gene delivery are given below:

- DNA/polymer complexation: Nanosize complex forms when cationic polymer neutralizes charged phosphate with negatively charged cell membrane.
- DNA/polymer complex: Also referred as polyplex, which passes through cell membrane by a nonspecific or receptor-mediated endocytosis.
- Endosome: Complex enters into cytoplasm through endosome.
- Transportation to nucleus.
- It is free to be encoded into a therapeutic protein or to be inserted into the genome [6, 8–10].

4. Targeted drug delivery

It is necessary to ensure that the nanomaterials are carefully delivered only to the infected region of the body without affecting the surrounding healthy tissues.

When drugs or gene-loaded nanoparticles are injected into bodies, they can circulate in the blood vessels by crossing the epithelial barriers before reaching the target site. Escape of nanoparticles from the vascular circulation occurs in either continuous or fenestrated tissues.

Nanoparticles can escape from the bloodstream at continuous vascular endothelium through paracellular pathway, intracellular process or transcellular pathway. It is different; the space between the fenestration sites on the endothelium is between 100 nm and 2 μm, which is longer than in healthy tissues that are normally 2–6 nm. Therefore, nanoparticles can penetrate fenestrations thus increase the drug concentration in target/tumor site which is called "enhanced permeation and retention effect (EPR effect)" [32–34]. Particle shape, surface charge, and feature are playing important roles in intercellular delivery [35, 36]. Quantity and type of polymers, particle size, solubility, biodegradability, and surface properties are having important role in release of bioactive drugs into the target site [37]. Drug entries through transcellular and paracellular pathways are shown in **Figure 1**.

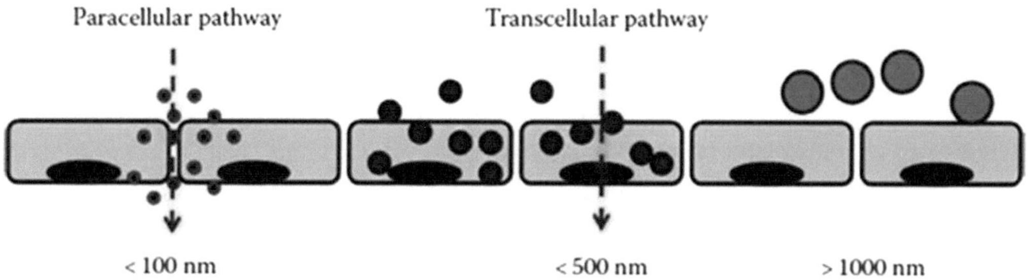

Figure 1. Drug entry through transcellular and paracellular pathways.

Targeted drug delivery is classified into two categories. They are

1. Passive targeting
2. Active targeting

4.1. Passive targeting

Passive targeting involves the cells that are to be targeted migrate toward the drug-carrying vehicles. This system is widely used in the delivery of cells like neutrophils, macrophages, dendritic cells for vaccination purposes. In this system, it is not necessary the drug-carrying vehicles in nanometer regime [38].

4.2. Active targeting

Active targeting involves rational design of nanosytems with suitable surface engineering performed with acceptable chemical linking strategies to specifically target the cell receptors of a target tissue. Furthermore, the targeting operates at two levels; first, the targeting of tissue/system in order to enrich the concentration of the carriers at the infected site [9, 39].

5. Nonviral vector gene delivery

Nonviral vector consists of either natural vectors (plasmid DNA or small nucleic acids, antisense oligonucleotides, small interfering RNAs) or synthetic vectors (liposomes, cationic polymers) [40]. Naked DNA, usually in plasmid form, is the simplest form of non-viral transferring of a gene into a target cell [41–44].

Nonviral vector delivery is categorized as organic (lipid complexes, conjugated polymers, cationic polymers, etc.) and inorganic systems (magnetic nanoparticles, quantum dots, carbon nanotubes, gold nanoparticles (GNPs), etc.) [45].

To achieve the desired therapeutic efficacy, a suitable carrier system is needed. Nanoparticles can be considered as a good carrier for various therapeutic applications due to the following reasons.

- They exist in the same size domain as proteins.
- They have large surface areas and ability to bind to a large number of surface functional groups.
- They possess controllable absorption and release properties and particle size and surface characteristics. [46].

6. Inorganic type nonviral delivery vectors

Inorganic type of nonviral delivery vectors are magnetic nanoparticles, quantum dots, and gold nanoparticles, and so on [31, 47].

6.1. Magnetic nanoparticle

Combination of inorganic nanoparticles with organic materials forms hybrids which possess unique physical, chemical, optical, and electrical properties. These unique properties can be utilized in different applications than large size materials. Recently, magnetic nanoparticles have been utilized as an effective tool in gene delivery because of its submicron size. Hence, much research has been carried out to control the size and shape of the metal nanostructure due to its magnetic, catalytic, electrical, and optical properties. Iron oxides, such as $CoFe_2O_4$, $NiFe_2O_4$, and $MnFe_2O_4$, exhibit superior performance compared to other magnetic materials but highly toxic to cells. The most widely used iron oxide as magnetic cores are magnetite (Fe_3O_4) and maghemite (γ-Fe_2O_3), possess high magnetic moments and relatively safe. The magnetic nanoparticle core is fairly reactive, prevents corrosion and leaking when applied *in vivo*. In the magnetic nanoparticle gene delivery system, the gene directly binds to the magnetic particle or carrier. In magnetic nanoparticle, a magnetic core is coated by a protective layer either by dispersing in a polymer matrix or encapsulated within a polymer/metallic shell, which can be combined with therapeutic agents (carrier/DNA complexes or other drugs) through covalent or noncovalent bond. Silica, gold, natural polymers, such as dextran, or synthetic polymers, such as PEI, PLL, PEG, and polyvinyl alcohol (PVA), are commonly used coating materials in magnetic nanoparticle. Introduction of various functional groups (organic linkers) like carboxyl, amines, thiols, and aldehyde can alter the surface properties to suit various therapeutic agents to improve targeted gene delivery. The preferred coating surface for magnetic particles is strongly cationic because of the negatively charged DNA molecules that are to be delivered. Magnetofection is a methodology based on the association of magnetic nanoparticle with gene vectors in order to optimize/enhance gene delivery in the presence of a magnetic field. The magnetic field is applied to move the MNP-gene vector complexes toward the target site. In magnetofection, gene can be delivered in few minutes to the target site, whereas traditional transfection methods can take several hours. Stability of any magnetic nanoparticles depends upon the balance between attractive (van der Waals and dipole-dipole) and repulsive (steric and electrostatic) forces between the particles and the surrounding solvent molecules. Temperature also has an effect in the stability of the magnetic nanoparticle due to energy transfer from the solvent molecules (Brownian motion) to the nanometric particles. Hence, magnetic nanoparticle can be coated with a biocompatible polymer to enhance its stability [30, 31, 48–62].

6.2. Metal nanoparticle (gold nanoparticle)

Owing to nano-dimension size to volume ratio and its stability, inorganic (metal) nanoparticles are being extensively used as promising gene carriers in various biomedical applications. Among the various metal nanoparticle gold nanoparticles (GNPs) are an obvious choice due to its inert, amenability of synthesis, high functionalization, fictionalization ability, higher absorption coefficient, good biocompatibility, less cytotoxic, ease of detection, and potential capability of targeted delivery, hence it is extensively used for various applications including drug and gene delivery. Due to its remarkable stability, large surface area, surface modification, and high biocompatibility, gold nanoparticles can retain the native structure and enzymatic activity of the attached proteins or enzymes in the drug delivery. Gold nanoparticles have large surface area due to which their surfaces are readily available for modification with targeting molecules or specific biomarkers and applicable in biomedical purposes.

Gold nanoparticles have large surface bio conjugation with molecular probes, and they also have many optical properties which are mainly concerned with localized plasmon resonance (PR). Gold nanoparticles can bind with a wide range of organic molecules and have tunable physical and chemical properties. Gold nanoparticles can be synthesized by chemical (seeding growth method), physical (γ-irradiation method, microwave irradiation method), and green methods (natural biomaterial egg shell membrane, sun light irradiation method).

Combination of gold nanoparticles into smart polymer like poly (N-isopropylacrylamine) is an effective process to enhance its properties. Gold nanoparticles exhibit different shapes such as spherical, sub-octahedral, octahedral, decahedral, icosahedral multiple twined, multiple twined, irregular shape, tetrahedral, nanotriangles, nanoprisms, hexagonal platelets, and nanorods, which are shown in **Figure 2**. Among the various shapes triangular-shaped nanoparticles show attractive optical properties compared with the spherical-shaped nanoparticles [30, 58, 63–72].

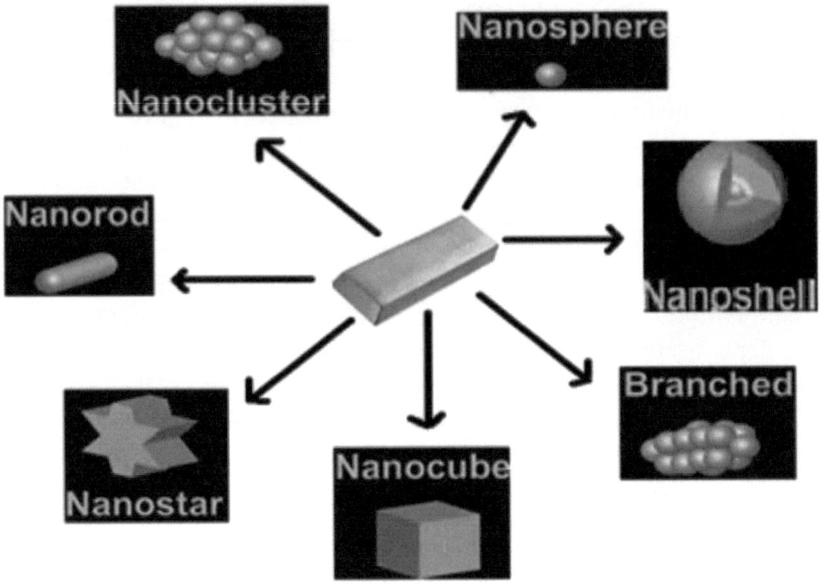

Figure 2. Various shapes of gold nanoparticle.

6.3. Quantum dots

Quantum dots are tiny semiconductor crystals of luminescent nanocrystals with rich surface chemistry and unique optical properties with the size of 1–10 nm made up of compounds from group II to VI and III to V, for example, Ag, Cd, Hg, Ln, P, Pb, Se, Te, Zn, and so on. QDs have distinctive characteristics such as size-tunable light emission, improved signal brightness, resistance against photobleaching, and simultaneous excitation of multiple fluorescence colors.

Depending on their size by laser, the quantum dots glow brightly in different colors, such as Adirondack Green (520nm), Blue (514 nm), Greenish blue (544 nm), Green (559 nm), Yellowish green (571 nm), Yellow (577 nm), Yellowish orange (581 nm), Fort Orange (600nm), Orange (610 nm), and Maple Red-Orange (620nm).

QDs are nearly spherical semiconductor particles with core-shell structure. Colloidal core/shell QDs, such as CdSe/ZnS, CdSe/CdS/ZnS, CdTe/CdSe, and InP/ZnS, are commonly synthesized for biomedical applications, whereas CdSe/ZnS, CdTe/ZnS, and CdSe/CdS/ZnS have been commonly used.

Quantum dots are made up of three parts, that is, core, shell, and cap.

Core is made up of CdSe, which is a semiconductor material. Core is surrounded by shell which is made up of ZnS for improving its optical properties and cap encapsulates the double layer quantum dots by different materials like silica which helps in improving solubility in aqueous buffers. Structure of quantum dot is shown in **Figure 3**.

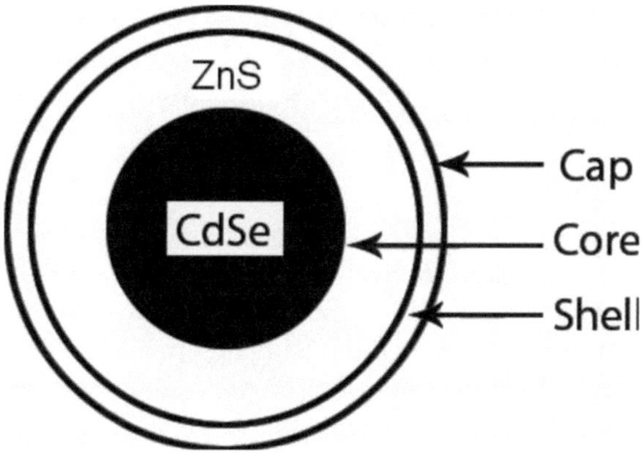

Figure 3. Structure of a quantum dot.

The semiconducting nature and the size-dependent fluorescence of these nanocrystals have been successfully applied for in vitro, in vivo transfection and for diagnosis of various diseases. One of the most important emerging applications of QDs appears to be *traceable* drug delivery, because it has the potential to elucidate the pharmacokinetics and pharmacodynamics of drug candidates and to provide the design principles for drug carrier engineering.

In gene technology, the quantum dot can be conjugated with oligonucleotide sequences (attached via surface carboxylic acid groups) may be targeted to bind with DNA or mRNA. Gene-associated drugs can be loaded within a QD core or attached to the surface of these nanoparticles through direct conjugation or electrostatic complexation by which QDs can protect the gene from degradation by nucleases. This property has been utilized for an assay of single nucleotide polymorphism (SNP). Due to concerns about long-term *in vivo* toxicity and degradation, QDs are currently limited to cell and small animal uses [30, 31, 77–101].

7. Conclusion

Recently nanotechnology-based gene delivery is one of the most attractive therapeutic methods for treatment of various diseases. In drug delivery, size and distribution of particles are critical parameters to target specific organs and tissues. Proteins (derived from their secondary structure) are suitable materials for drug/gene carriers due to their precise molecular sizes. An ideal nanoparticle formulation for a drug or gene carrier system can achieve long circulation time, low immunogenicity, good biocompatibility, and selective targeting.

Gene delivery involves viral and non-viral vectors. Viral vectors are having low loading capacity, large-scale manufacturing, quality control cost, and safety factor such as immunogenicity and potential oncogenicity. From the stability and safety concern, non-viral vectors have more efficiently passing the gene transfection through the biological barriers compared to viral vectors. Organic, inorganic, and various hybrid materials are used for the preparation of nanoparticles. Among these, polymeric nanoparticles have great therapeutic application due to its wide range of sizes and varieties and can be used in sustained and targeted gene delivery for long periods. Biopolymers used for the preparation of nonviral vectors possess several favorable characteristics, such as high biocompatibility, low toxicity, good biodegradability, and abundant renewable sources, which can be used for efficiency delivery of drug/gene to the target site.

Choosing a suitable design of nanoparticle structure can increase gene transfection efficiency to overcome extracellular and intracellular transfection barriers: the blood stream, the cellular membrane, endosomes, and the nuclear membrane. Nanoparticle in gene delivery depends upon the nature of the polymer charge and its chain length. Furthermore, modifications in the nanoparticle by introducing ligands onto the surface can enhance localization and retention in specific target tissue, local delivery of agents to a large volume of tissues for better clinical application. However, biopolymer-based nanoparticle will become a tool in near future for the precisely targeted delivery of drugs and genes in many therapeutic fields, but toxicological issues and degradation products of nanoparticles are need to be considered before being applied into humans.

Author details

Sakthivel Lakshmana Prabu[1*], Timmadonu Narasimman Kuppusami Suriyaprakash[2] and Rathinasabapathy Thirumurugan[3]

*Address all correspondence to: slaxmanvel@gmail.com

1 Department of Pharmaceutical Technology, Bharathidasan Institute of Technology, Anna University, Tiruchirapalli, Tamilnadu, India

2 Dept of Pharmaceutics, Al Shifa College of Pharmacy, Kerala

3 School of Pharmacy, International Medical University, Malaysia

References

[1] Fattal E, Barratt G. Nanotechnologies and controlled release systems for delivery and antisense oligonucleotides and small interfering RNA. Br. J. Pharmacol. 2009; 157(2): 179–194.

[2] Erdal C, Ali DS, Emre SC. Gene delivery systems: recent progress in viral and non-viral therapy. In: Recent Advances in Novel Drug Carrier Systems, Ali DS, ed. Croatia, InTech, 2012. DOI: 10.5772/53392. http://www.intechopen.com/books/recent-advances-in-novel-drug-carrier-systems/gene-delivery-systems-recent-progress-in-viral-and-non-viral-therapy

[3] Kaul G, Amiji M. Tumor-targeted gene delivery using poly-(ethylene glycol)-modified gelatin nanoparticles: in vitro and in vivo studies. Pharm. Res. 2005; 22(6): 951–961.

[4] Durland RH, Eastman EM. Manufacturing and quality control of plasmid-based gene expression systems. Adv. Drug Deliv. Rev. 1998; 30: 33–48.

[5] Labhasetwar V, Chen B, Muller DWM, Bonadio J, Ciftci K, March K, et al. Gene-based therapies for restenosis. Adv. Drug Deliv. Rev. 1997; 24:109–20.

[6] Jordan M. Synthetic and semisynthetic polymers as vehicles for in vitro gene delivery into cultured mammalian cells. In: Synthetic Polymers for Biotechnology and Medicine, Freitag R, ed. Georgetown, DC: Eurekah.com/Landes Bioscience, 2003; pp. 19–39.

[7] Langer R. Introduction. In: Polymeric Gene Delivery: Principles and Applications, Amiji MM, ed. Boca Raton, FL: Taylor & Francis, 2005; pp. 1–2.

[8] Luten J, Van Nostruin CF, De Smedt SC, Hennink WE. Biodegradable polymers as nonviral carriers for plasmid DNA delivery. J Control. Release. 2008; 126(2): 97–110.

[9] Merdan T, Kopecek J, Kissel T. Prospects for cationic polymers in gene and oligonucleotide therapy against cancer. Adv. Drug Deliv. Rev. 2002; 54(5): 715–758.

[10] Wong SY, Pelet JM, Putnam D. Polymer systems for gene delivery-past, present, and future. Prog. Poly. Sci. 2007; 32(8–9):799–837.

[11] Raftery R, O'Brien FJ, Cryan SA. Chitosan for gene delivery and orthopedic tissue engineering applications. Molecules. 2013; 18: 5611–5647.

[12] Rana TM. Illuminating the silence: Understanding the structure and function of small RNAs. Nat. Rev. Mol. Cell Biol. 2007; 8: 23–36.

[13] Guo P, Coban O, Snead NM, Trebley J, Hoeprich S, Guo S, et al. Engineering RNA for targeted siRNA delivery and medical application. Adv. Drug Deliv. Rev. 2010; 62: 650–666.

[14] Van Rooij E. The art of microRNA research. Circ. Res. 2011; 108: 219–234.

[15] Jin L, Zeng X, Liu M, Deng Y, He N. Current progress in gene delivery technology based on chemical methods and nano-carriers. Theranostics. 2014; 4(3): 240–255.

[16] Putnam D. Polymers for gene delivery across length scales. Nat. Mater. 2006; 5: 439–451.

[17] Pack DW, Hoffman AS, Pun S, Stayton PS. Design and development of polymers for gene delivery. Nat. Rev. Drug Discov. 2005; 4: 581–593.

[18] Mansouri S, Lavigne P, Corsi K, Benderdour M, Beaumont E, Fernandes JC. Chitosan-DNA nanoparticles as nonviral vectors in gene therapy: strategies to improve transfection efficacy. Eur. J Pharm. Biopharm. 2004; 57: 1–8.

[19] Yang Y, Li Q, Erte HCJ, Wilson JM. Cellular and humoral immune responses to viral antigens create barriers to lung directed gene therapy with recombinant adenoviruses. J Virol. 1995; 69: 2004–2015.

[20] Giannoukakis N, Thomson A, Robbins P. Gene therapy in transplantation. Gene Ther. 1999; 6(9): 1499–1511.

[21] Liu F, Liang KW, Huang L. Systemic administration of naked DNA: Gene transfer to skeletal muscle. Mol. Interv. 2001; 1(3): 168–172.

[22] Mahato RI. Non-viral peptide-based approaches to gene delivery. J. Drug Target. 1999; 7(4): 249–268.

[23] Itaka K, Kataoka K. Recent development of nonviral gene delivery systems with virus-like structures and mechanisms. Eur. J Pharm. Biopharm. 2009; 71: 475–483.

[24] Mrsny RJ. Tissue- and cell-specific targeting for the delivery of genetic information. In: Polymeric Gene Delivery: Principles and Applications, Amiji MM, ed. Boca Raton, FL: Taylor & Francis, 2005; pp. 4–30.

[25] Lee M, Kim SW. Polyethylene glycol-conjugated copolymers for plasmid DNA delivery. Pharm. Res. 2005; 22(1): 1–10.

[26] Nomura T, Koreeda N, Yamashita F, Takakura Y, Hashida M. Effect of particle size and charge on the disposition of lipid carriers after intratumoral injection into tissue-isolated tumors. Pharm. Res. 1998; 15(1): 128–132.

[27] Liang GF, Zhu YL, Sun B, Hu FH, Tian T, Li SC, et al. PLGA-based gene delivering nanoparticle enhance suppression effect of miRNA in HePG2 cells. Nanoscale Res. Lett. 2011; 6: 447.

[28] Jin S, Ye K. Mediated drug delivery and gene therapy. Biotechnol. Prog. 2007; 23: 32–41.

[29] Nitta SK, Numata K. Biopolymer-based nanoparticles for drug/gene delivery and tissue engineering. Int. J. Mol. Sci. 2013; 14: 1629-1654.

[30] Zhang X, Balazs DA, Godbey WT. Nanobiomaterials for nonviral gene delivery. In: Nanobiomaterials Handbook, Sitharaman B, ed. Taylor & Francis: CRC press, 2011; pp. 13–1 to 13–25.

[31] Dizaj SM, Jafari S, Khosroushahi AY. A sight on the current nanoparticle-based gene delivery vectors. Nanoscale Res. Lett. 2014, 9: 252.

[32] Adiseshaiah PP, Hall JB, McNeil SE. Nanomaterial standards for efficacy and toxicity assessment. Wiley Interdiscip. Rev. 2010; 2: 99–112.

[33] Gaumet M, Vargas A, Gurny R, Delie F. Nanoparticles for drug delivery: The need for precision in reporting particle size parameters. Eur. J. Pharm. Biopharm. 2008; 69: 1–9.

[34] Maeda H, Wu J, Sawa T, Matsumura Y, Hori K. Tumor vascular permeability and the EPR effect in macromolecular therapeutics: a review. J. Control. Release 2000; 65: 271–284.

[35] Mizrahy S, Peer D. Polysaccharides as building blocks for nanotherapeutics. Chem. Soc. Rev. 2012; 41: 2623–2640.

[36] Petros RA, DeSimone JM. Strategies in the design of nanoparticles for therapeutic applications. Nat. Rev. Drug Discov. 2010; 9: 615–627.

[37] Mohanraj V, Chen Y. Nanoparticles-A Review. Tropical J. Pharm. Res. 2006; 5; 561–573.

[38] Hedley ML, Curley J, Urban R. Microspheres containing plasmid-encoded antigens elicit cytotoxic T-cell responses. Nat. Med. 1998; 4: 365–368.

[39] Hermanson G. Bioconjugate Techniques. Academic Press Inc., San Diego, CA, 1996; pp. 570–592.

[40] Lu Y. Transcriptionally regulated, prostate-targeted gene therapy for prostate cancer. Adv. Drug Deliv. Rev. 2009; 61(7–8): 572–588.

[41] Conwell CC, Huang L. Recent advances in nonμviral gene delivery. Adv. Genet. 2005; 53:1–18.

[42] Niidome T, Huang L. Gene therapy progress and prospects: nonviral vectors. Gene Ther. 2002; 9(24):1647–1652.

[43] Bigger BW, Tolmachov O, Collombet JM, Fragkos M, Palaszewski I, Coutelle C. An araC-controlled bacterial cre expression system to produce DNA minicircle vectors for nuclear and mitochondrial gene therapy. J Biol. Chem. 2001; 276(25):23018–23027.

[44] Mayrhofer P, Schleef M, Jechlinger W. Use of minicircle plasmids for gene therapy. Methods Mol. Biol. 2009, 542: 87–104.

[45] Lee JM, Yoon TJ, Cho YS. Recent developments in nanoparticle-based siRNA delivery for cancer therapy. Biomed Res. Int. 2013; 782041.

[46] Nitta SK, Numata K. Biopolymer-based nanoparticles for drug/gene delivery and tissue engineering. Int. J. Mol. Sci. 2013; 14(1):1629–1654.

[47] Lee JM, Yoon TJ, Cho YS. Recent developments in nanoparticle-based siRNA delivery for cancer therapy. Biomed Res Int. 2013; 2013:782041. Doi: 10.1155/2013/782041.

[48] Athar M, Das AJ. Therapeutic nanoparticle: State of the art of Nanomedicine. Adv. Mater. Rev. 2014; 1(1): 25–37.

[49] Lubbe AS, Alexiou C, Bergemann C. Clinical applications of magnetic drug targeting. J Surg. Res. 2001; 95: 200–206.

[50] Scherer F, Anton M, Schillinger U, Henke J, Bergemann C, Krüger A, et al. Magnetofection: enhancing and targeting gene delivery by magnetic force in vitro and in vivo. Gene Ther. 2002; 9: 102–109.

[51] Plank C, Zelphati O, Mykhaylyk O. Magnetically enhanced nucleic acid delivery. Ten years of magnetofection - Progress and prospects. Adv. Drug. Deliv. Rev. 2011; 63(14–15): 1300–1303.

[52] Scherer F, Plank C. Magnetofection: Using magnetic particles and magnetic force to enhance and to target nucleic acid delivery. In: Smyth Templeton N, ed. Gene and Cell Therapy: Therapeutic Mechanisms and Strategies; 3rd Ed. Boca Raton, FL: CRC Press 2009; pp. 379–404.

[53] McBain SC, Yiu HHP, Dobson J. Magnetic nanoparticles for gene and drug delivery. Int. J. Nanomed. 2008; 3(2): 169–180.

[54] Buerli T, Pellegrino C, Baer K, Lardi-Studler B, Chudotvorova I, Fritschy JM, et al. Efficient transfection of DNA or shRNA vectors into neurons using magnetofection. Nat. Protoc. 2007; 2: 3090–101.

[55] Xenariou S, Griesenbach U, Ferrari S, Dean P, Scheule RK, Cheng SH, et al. Using magnetic forces to enhance non-viral gene transfer to airway epithelium in vivo. Gene Ther. 2006; 13: 1545–52.

[56] Fernandez- Pacheco R, Valdivia JG, Ibarra MR. Magnetic nanoparticles for local drug delivery using magnetic implants. Meth. Mol. Biol. 2009; 544: 559–69.

[57] McBain SC, Yiu HHP, Dobson J. Magnetic nanoparticles for gene and drug delivery. Int. J. Nanomed. 2008; 3(2): 169–180.

[58] Xu ZP, Zeng QH, Lu GQ, Yu AB. Inorganic nanoparticles as carriers for efficient cellular delivery. Chem. Eng. Sci. 2006; 61(3):1027–1040.

[59] Arruebo M, Pacheco RF, Ibarra MR, Santamaria J. Magnetic nanoparticle for drug delivery. Nano Today. 2007; 2(3): 22–32.

[60] Krotz F, de Wit C, Sohn HY, Zahler S, Gloe T, Pohl U, et al. Magnetofection:a highly efficient tool for antisense oligonucleotide delivery in vitro and in vivo. Mol. Ther. 2003; 7(5 Pt 1): 700–710.

[61] Krotz F, Sohn HY, Gloe T, Plank C, Pohl U. Magnetofection potentiates gene delivery to cultured endothelial cells. J. Vasc. Res. 2003; 40(5): 425–434.

[62] Kamau SW, Hassa PO, Hottiger MO. Enhancement of the efficiency of non-viral gene delivery by application of pulsed magnetic field. Nucleic Acids Res. 2006; 34(5): e40.

[63] Tiwari PK, Lee YS. Gene delivery in conjunction with gold nanoparticle and tumor treating electric field. J. Appl. Phys. 2013; 114(5): 054902.

[64] Alanazi AK, Radwan AA, Alsarra IA. Biopharmaceutical applications of nanogold. Saudi Pharm. J. 2010; 18: 179–193.

[65] Di Guglielmo C, Lopez DR, De Lapuente J, Mallafre JM, Suarez MB. Embryotoxicity of cobalt ferrite and gold nanoparticles: a first in vitro approach. Reprod. Toxicol. 2010; 30: 271–276.

[66] Kim D, Jon S. Gold nanoparticles in image-guided cancer therapy. Inorg. Chim. Acta. 2012; 393: 154–164.

[67] Stobiecka M, Hepel M. Double-shell gold nanoparticle-based DNA-carriers with poly-L-lysine binding surface. Biomaterials. 2011; 32: 3312–3321.

[68] Chithrani DB, Dunne M, Stewart J, Allen C, Jaffray DA. Cellular uptake and transport of gold nanoparticles incorporated in a liposomal carrier. Nanomed. Nanotechnol. Biol. Med. 2010; 6: 161–169.

[69] Giljohann DA, Seferos DS, Daniel WL, Massich MD, Patel PC, Mirkin CA. Gold nanoparticles for biology and medicine. Angewandte Chem. 2010; 49: 3280–3294.

[70] Papasani MR, Wang G, Hill RA. Gold nanoparticles: the importance of physiological principles to devise strategies for targeted drug delivery. Nanomed. Nanotechnol. Biol. Med. 2012; 8: 804–814.

[71] Ghosh R, Singh LC, Shohet JM, Gunaratne PH. A gold nanoparticle platform for the delivery of functional microRNAs into cancer cells. Biomaterials. 2013; 34: 807–816.

[72] Pissuwan D, Niidome T, Cortie MB. The forthcoming applications of gold nanoparticles in drug and gene delivery systems. J Con. Rel. 2011; 149: 65–71.

[73] Khan MS, Vishakante GD, Siddaramaiah H. Gold nanoparticles: a paradigm shift in biomedical applications. Adv. Colloid Interface Sci. 2013; 199–200: 44–58.

[74] Tarnawski R, Ulbricht M. Amphiphilic gold nanoparticles: Synthesis, characterization and adsorption to PEGylated polymer surfaces. Colloid Surface A: Physicochem. Engineer Aspects. 2011; 374: 13–21.

[75] Benkovicova M, Vegso K, Siffalovic P, Jergel M, Luby S, Majkova E. Preparation of gold nanoparticles for plasmonic applications. Thin Solid Films. 2013; 543:138–141.

[76] Khan AK, Rashid R, Murtaza G, Zahra A. Gold Nanoparticles: synthesis and applications in drug delivery. Trop. J Pharm. Res. 2014; 13(7): 1169–1177.

[77] Probst CE, Zrazhevskiy P, Bagalkot V, Gao X. Quantum dots as a platform for nanoparticle drug delivery vehicle design. Adv. Drug Deliv. Rev. 2013; 65(5): 703–718.

[78] Derfus AM, Chen AA, Bhatia SN, et al. Targeted quantum dot conjugates for siRNA delivery. Bioconjug. Chem. 2007; 18(5): 1391–1396.

[79] Qi L, Gao X. Emerging application of quantum dots for drug delivery and therapy. Expert Opin. Drug Deliv. 2008; 5(3): 263–267.

[80] Gulia S, Kakkar R. ZnO quantum dots for biomedical applications. Adv. Mater. Lett. 2013; 4(12): 876–887.

[81] Chen AA, Derfus AM, Khetani SA, Bhatia SN. Quantum dots to monitor RNAi delivery and improve gene silencing. Nucleic Acids Res. 2005; 33(22): e190.

[82] Dabbousi BO, Viejo RJ, Mikulec FV, Heine JR, Mattoussi H, Ober R, et al., (CdSe)ZnS core-shell quantum dots: synthesis and characterization of a size series of highly luminescent nanocrystallites. J. Phys. Chem. B. 1997; 101: 9463–9475.

[83] Modani S, Kharwade M, Nijhawan M. Quantum dots: a novelty of medical field with multiple applications. Int. J. Curr. Pharm. Res. 2013; 5(4): 55–59.

[84] Dey NS, Rao MEB. Quantum Dot: novel carrier for drug delivery. Int. J Res. Pharm. Biomed. Sci.2011; 2(2): 448–458.

[85] Rathore KS, Lowalekar R, Nema RK. Quantum dots: a future drug delivery system. Pharma Rev. 2006; 4: 30–32.

[86] Ghasemi Y, Peymanib P, Afifi S. Quantum dot: magic nanoparticle for imaging, detection and targeting. Acta Biomed. 2009; 80: 156–165.

[87] Patel HR. Quantum dots: a novel technique for drug delivery and therapy 2007; available at http://www.pharmainfo.net/reviews/quantum-dots-novel-technique-drug-delivery-and-therapy. Accessed on 10 September 2014.

[88] Pandurangan DK, Mounika KS. Quantum dot aptamers: an emerging technology with wide scope in pharmacy. Int. J Pharm. Pharm. Sci. 2012; 4(3):24–31.

[89] Genger UR, Grabolle M, Jaricot SC, Nitschke R, Nann T. Quantum dots versus organic dyes as fluorescent labels. Nat. Methods 2008; 5(9):763–775.

[90] Mishra S, Tripathy P, Sinha SP. Advancements in the field of quantum dots. Int. J. Adv/ Res. Tech. 2012; 1(3): 1–5.

[91] Jamiesona T, Bakhshi R, Petrovaa D, Pococka R, Imanib M, Seifaliana AM. Biological applications of quantum dots. Biomaterials. 2007; 28: 4717–4732.

[92] Drbohlavova J, Adam V, Kizek R, Hubalek J. Quantum dots: characterization, preparation and usage in biological systems. Int .J Mol. Sci. 2009;10:656–673.

[93] http://www.americanelements.com/quantum-dots.html

[94] Zrazhevskiyn P, Gao X. Multifunctional quantum dots for personalized medicine. Nano Today 2009; 4(5): 414–428.

[95] Wang Y, Chen L, Quantum dots, lighting up the research and development of nanomedicine. Nanomed: Nanotech. Biol. Med. 2011; 7: 385–402.

[96] Vengala P, Dasari A, Yeruva N, Quantum dots for drug delivery and therapy international. J Pharm. Tech. 2012; 4(2): 2055–2074.

[97] Mukherjee S, Das U, Quantum dots: an optimistic approach to novel therapeutics. Int. J . Pharm. Sci. Rev. Res. 2011; 7: 59–64.

[98] Cheki M, Moslehi M, Assadi M. Marvelous applications of quantum dots. Eur. Rev. Med. Pharmacol. Sci. 2013; 17: 1141–1148.

[99] Ozkan M. Quantum dots and other nanoparticles: what can they offer to drug discoveryμ Drug Discov. Today. 2004; 9: 1065–1071.

[100] Dorfs D, Krahne R, Falqui A, Manna L, Giannini C, Zanchet D. Quantum Dots: Synthesis and Characterization. In: Comprehensive Nanoscience and Technology, David LA, Gregory DS, Gary PW, eds. Amsterdam: Academic Press; pp. 219–270.

[101] Mokari T, Banin U. Synthesis and properties of CdSe/ZnS core/shell nanorods. Chem. Mater. 2003; 15: 3955–3960.

Chapter 3

Lipid-Based Nano-Delivery for Oral Administration of Poorly Water Soluble Drugs (PWSDs): Design, Optimization and *in vitro* Assessment

Mohsin Kazi

Additional information is available at the end of the chapter

http://dx.doi.org/10.5772/65710

Abstract

Currently, more than 90% of compounds identified are water insoluble and or poorly water soluble, which is a bottle neck in the development of many new drug candidates. These poorly soluble drug molecules are difficult to formulate using conventional approaches and are associated with numerous formulation-related performance issues. Formulating these compounds using lipid-based systems is one of the rapidly growing interests and suitable drug delivery strategies. Lipid formulations such as self-emulsifying/microemulsifying/nanoemulsifying drug delivery systems (SEDDS/SMEDDS/SNEDDS) have been attempted in many researches to improve the bioavailability and dissolution rate for their better dispersion properties. One of the greatest advantages of incorporating the poorly soluble drug into such formulation products is their spontaneous emulsion and or microemulsion/nanoemulsion formation in aqueous media. The performance and ongoing advances in manufacturing technologies have rapidly introduced lipid-based drug formulations as commercial products into the marketplace with several others in clinical development. The current chapter aims to present the characteristics feature, development and utilization of oral lipid-based nanoformulations within the drug delivery regime. The content of the chapter also provides an insight into the *in vitro* evaluation of lipid-based nanosystems and their limitations.

Keywords: lipid-based formulation, self-nanoemulsifying drug delivery systems (SNEDDS), poorly water soluble drugs (PWSDs), lipid formulation classification systems (LFCS), solubility enhancement

1. Introduction

Due to the continuous rise in the number of low solubility drug molecules and lack of more targeted drug therapies, the drug development has become more complex and challenging job within the industry. In fact, up to 90% of today's drug candidates are suffering from low aqueous solubility, which is commonly associated with low bioavailability, high intra- and inter-subject variability and lack of dose suitability [1, 2]. In keeping these challenges in mind, drug formulators must seek new techniques and innovative formulation approaches to overcome such hurdles and ensure effective treatments for the patients in need.

It is more than a decade, when lipid-based formulations have been considered as a well-established strategy for improving oral bioavailability and minimizing variable food effect of poorly soluble compounds. Lipids have been used as carriers in various delivery systems for drug administration, including solutions, suspensions, emulsions, and more attractively self-emulsifying/microemulsifying/nanoemulsifying drug delivery systems (SEDDS/SMEDDS/SNEDDS) that are designed to increase solubility and bioavailability of drugs belonging to the BCS Class II–IV [3]. Among several approaches, which are currently available to incorporate active pharmaceutical drugs into lipid vehicles in a variety of dosage forms, SEDDS, SMEDDS and or SNEDDS have proved to be the most successful approaches in improving the bioavailability [4]. The initial key achievement of these formulation systems (SEDDS/SMEDDS/SNEDDS) is to increase the solubilization of the poorly water soluble drugs (PWSDs) by the formation of emulsions and or micellar systems (colloidal solutions).

These systems advantageously present the drug in solubilized form, and their relatively smaller droplet sizes provide a large interfacial area enhancing the activity of pancreatic lipase to hydrolyze triglycerides and thereby promoting faster drug release containing mixed micelles of bile salts. The development of Neoral® (cyclosporin A) as a commercial product exhibits an excellent example of the utilization of these systems [5].

Nanotechnology has become a buzzword for scientific experts, and efforts are ongoing to extend its applications in various medical and pharmaceutical aspects. The nanoscale technologies can be generally categorized into: lipid-based nanocarriers, polymeric nanocarriers, inorganic nanocarriers, and drug nanoparticles or nanosuspensions [6]. Within the lipid-based nanocarriers category, there has been a resurgence of interest in nanoemulsions since low energy emulsification methods, such as spontaneous or self-nanoemulsification, have been developed. SNEDDS are anhydrous homogenous liquid mixtures, composing oil, surfactant, drug and/or cosolvents, which spontaneously form transparent nanoemulsion (20–250 nm droplet size) upon aqueous dilution with mild agitation [6, 7].

Being nanosized, SNEDDS offer a strong alternative to the more conventional oral formulations of lipophilic compounds. SNEDDS introduce the drug in solution within nanosized oil droplets. These fine droplets are emptied rapidly from the stomach resulting in faster drug release all over the gastrointestinal (GI) tract. An additional advantage of SNEDDS over simple oily solutions is granting much larger interfacial area for partitioning of the drug between oil and water leading to ease of dispersibility [8]. In contrast to oily solutions, SNEDDS does not depend on the action of bile salts, enzymes and/or other effects related to the (fed/fasted) state of the stomach [9]. Thus, SNEDDS can reduce the variability in rate and extent of absorption and grant more reproducible plasma concentration levels [10].

Compared with conventional nanoemulsions, SNEDDS can offer the advantages of improved physical and/or chemical stability of the formulation and ability to fill them into unit dosage forms, such as soft/hard capsules, which improve their commercial viability, patient compliance/tolerability and reduce palatability-related concerns [6]. A key feature of a successful SNEDDS formulation is its capability to hold the drug in solution, throughout the GIT, for sufficient time to allow for absorption [11]. Many PWSDs have high solubility in SNEDDS formulations but could make a risk of precipitation after aqueous dispersion of the formulation or during its digestion in the intestine [12].

The current chapter will provide all the information to probe factors which influence the selection of successful lipid nanoformulations and affect the fate of the PWSDs after oral administration. The investigational research presented in this chapter will also provide additional information regarding current practice of lipid formulations with a particular emphasis on self-nanoemulsifying drug delivery systems (SNEDDS), the trends and perspectives and the fate of PWSDs formulated in SNEDDS.

2. Lipid nanoformulations: design approach

Lipid excipients are comprised of a large group of physically and chemically diverse glycerides, which may be used in simple (single oil solutions of the drug substance) or in more complex nanocarriers (SMEDDS/SNEDDS, drug dissolved in the mixture of glyceride, surfactant and or cosolvent), with considerable flexibility in formulation design [12].

Simple oil formulations are generally composed of mono-, di-, or triglycerides or their derivatives and differ on the content of medium- (C_6-C_{10} in chain length) or long-chain (C_{12}-C_{24} in chain length) fatty acids. Glyceride esters are water immiscible, and their solvent capacities for drug substances vary according to the fatty acid chain length. Many lipid excipients (oils, surfactants), which are regarded as acceptable food grade materials, expected to be well tolerated by the body [13], even as parenteral emulsion dosage form [14]. These excipients have a history of use in a wide variety of pharmaceuticals.

In simple terms, lipid nanoformulations can be distinguished according to their dispersion and digestion in the aqueous content of the gut [15, 16]. Emulsion droplet size has been considered to be an important part in the performance of self-nanoemulsifying systems since particle size can determine the rate and extent of drug release *in vitro* [17]. However, the relative digestion rate would be expected to vary if the formulation is modified, and the critical factor is the fate of the drug after digestion of the formulation, in particular whether or not the drug remains in a solubilized state.

Function	Composition and description	Commercial name	Supplier
Oil	**Medium-chain triglycerides (C_8-C_{10}):** Fractionated coconut oil and palm seed oil, triglycerides of caprylic/capric acid	Miglyol 812, 810, Capmul MCM, Captex 355, etc.	Gattefosse corporation, France; Abitec Corp., Janesville, USA; Sasol GmbH, Witten, Germany; Nikko Chemicals Co., Tokyo, Japan; **Cremer Oleo GmbH & Co. KG,** Hamburg, Germany; Lipoid, Germany; BASF Co., Germany
	Long-chain triglycerides (C_{14}-C_{22}): Vegetable oils are glyceride esters of mixed unsaturated long-chain fatty acids, commonly known as long-chain triglycerides	Soybean oil, sesame oil, corn oil, olive oil, peanut oil, cottonseed oil, rapeseed oil, etc.	
	Mixed mono-, di- and triglycerides: Novel semisynthetic medium- and long-chain derivatives. Esters of propylene glycol and mixture of mono- and diglycerides of caprylic/capric acid	Imwitor 988, Imwitor 308, Maisene 35-1, etc.	
	Polar oil: Some excipients which are traditionally thought of as hydrophobic surfactants, such as sorbitan fatty acid esters	Span 80, 85, etc.	
Nonionic surfactant	**Water insoluble:** Oleate esters, such as polyoxyethylene (20) sorbitan trioleate, PEG-6-sorbitan oleate and polyoxyethylene (25) glyceryl trioleate are commonly used in the pharmaceutical industries	Polysorbate 85 (Tween 85), TO-106 V, Tagat TO, etc.	
	Water soluble: The popular castor oil derivatives with saturated alkyl chains resulting from hydrogenation of materials derived from a vegetable oil. Other derivatives include polysorbate 80 which are predominantly ether ethoxylates and phospholipids	Cremophor RH40, Cremophor EL, HCO30, Tween 20, 80, poloxamer 407, various Labrasols, Labrafac Labrafils, Gelucires, Soy phosphatidylcholine, etc.	
Cosolvent	The most popular water soluble cosolvents are propylene glycol, polyethylene glycol, ethanol and glycerol. Others are diethylene glycol monoethyl ether, propylene carbonate, tetrahydrofurfuryl alcohol, polyethylene glycol ether	PG, PEG 300, PEG 400, 600, transcutol, glycofurol, etc.	
Other excipient	Many oil-soluble antioxidants	α-Tocopherol, β-carotene, butylated hydroxytoluene (BHT), butylated hydroxyanisole (BHA), propyl gallate, ascorbyl palmitate, etc.	

Table 1. Common excipients for designing self-nanoemulsifying formulations and the list of their suppliers.

2.1. Excipients used to design lipid-based nanoformulations

Excipients play a key role in designing successful nanoformulations with a sound control strategy and influence business-critical and clinically significant drug product performance outcomes such as stability, bioavailability and manufacturability. The design of lipid-based nanoformulations, particularly SNEDDS, is comparatively simple as the drug need to be incorporated into a suitable oil-surfactant mixture, which could be filled in a soft or hard gelatin capsules. Various choices of lipid excipients are available in the market. Numerous lipids are amphiphilic in nature, which contain both hydrophilic and lipophilic portions (fatty acid) [18]. The morphology of the lipids should be assessed as melting point increases when the length of fatty acid chain increases, but it decreases when unsaturation of the fatty acid increases [19]. Choice of excipients for successfully designed lipid-based nanocarriers is determined based on factors, such as miscibility; solvent capacity; self-dispersibility; digestibility; irritancy; toxicity; purity; chemical stability; compatibility with capsule; melting point; and cost. Since these excipients can affect the drugs bioavailability, it is necessary to identify the characteristics of these excipients. Details of the lipids (oils, nonionic surfactants, cosolvents), their compositions and list of suppliers are given in **Table 1**.

3. Lipid nanocarriers and recent advancements in oral drug delivery

Lipid-based nanoformulations as drug delivery vehicles signify a promising strategy that incorporates or encapsulates the drug molecules and are biodegradable or biocompatible. They are containing nanosized droplets typically ranging from 0 to 250 nm [20]. The entrapped drug molecules can be taken intact and protected against degradation by gastrointestinal (GI) fluids, while drug absorption through the GI epithelium or lymphatic transport can be enhanced. Possible mechanisms of transport of these nanocarriers across GI mucosa are introduced later in the chapter. These focus on effects of size and surface properties of the nanocarriers on the nonspecific or targeted uptake by enterocytes and/or M cells. Applications of various oral nanocarrier formulations, such as lipid nanoparticles and SMEDDS/SNEDDS, are reviewed in several recent publications [4, 21, 22]. **Figure 1** shows an encapsulated SNEDDS designed for oral administration, which are the most efficient formulations for improving the apparent aqueous solubility of PWSDs.

Within the scope of the current chapter, the most advanced SNEDDS and/or SMEDDS systems have been explored as potential nanocarriers, which are much more stable kinetically and thermodynamically and showed great potential for improving the bioavailability of orally administered drugs. In a pure drug nanoparticle formulation, submicron size particles of drugs are stabilized in aqueous medium with generally regarded as safe (GRAS) listed excipients blend. Such formulation can be used for drugs with poor solubility in water and oil, high melting point, high log *P* and high dose.

When saquinavir (HIV protease inhibitor) in 1995 was marketed for the first time as mesylate salt formulation in a hard gelatin capsule (Invirase®), its bioavailability was only 4% and highly variable [23]. Later on, after 2 years, a self-nanoemulsifying formulation of saquinavir (Fortovase®) containing medium-chain mono- and diglycerides, povidone and α-tocopherol was able to increase bioavailability threefold higher than Invirase® in humans [23, 24]. Several other published [10, 25, 26] and unpublished case studies are also available that established the significance of rational approach in designing SMEDDS/SNEDDS which can improve the *in vivo* absorption of the PWSDs. The commercial product such as amprenavir (agenerase), ciprofloxacin (cipro), fenofibrate (fenogal), liponavir/ritonavir (kaletra, norvir), etc., have been formulated using suitable SMEDDS/SNEDDS [24, 27].

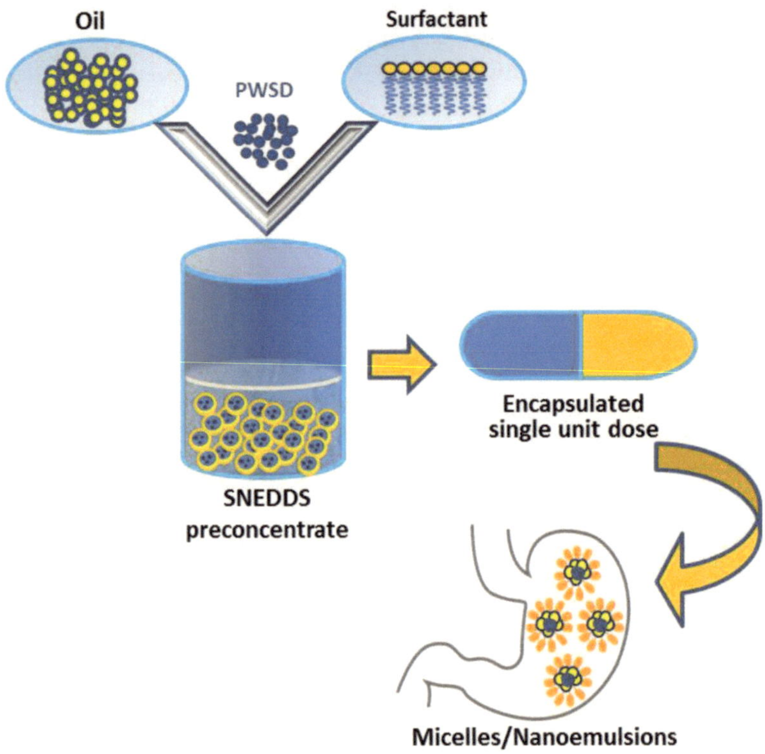

Figure 1. The encapsulated SNEDDS designed for oral administration of PWSDs. *Adapted with permission from Ref. [21].

4. Concept of nanoemulsions within lipid-based formulation

The potentiality of nanoemulsions within lipid-based drug delivery systems was explored almost four decades ago. In simple term, nanoemulsions are the emulsions comprising nanosized droplets and they are well dispersed, transparent and kinetically stable for several months. Their physical stability can be improved by careful selection of surfactants and the ratio of oil/water/surfactant and also the efficiency of equipment used to reduce droplet sizes.

Not only for oral delivery, nanoemulsions are used as greater transmucosal and transdermal drug delivery vehicles due to their remarkable wetting, spreading and penetration abilities.

4.1. SMEDDS vs SNEDDS

SMEDDS and SNEDDS are almost similar lipid dosage form which can be prepared from same materials comprising a simple mixture of oils, surfactants and possibly cosolvents. SMEDDS have the ability to form fine oil in water (O/W) microemulsion, and SNEDDS produce nanoemulsion upon mild agitation in the presence of an aqueous (preferably intestinal) media [28]. The structure provides both SMEDDS and SNEDDS as good candidates for oral delivery of PWSDs with adequate solubility in oil only or oil/surfactant blends and establishes the desired reproducible pharmacokinetic profile. Upon dilution, SMEDDS form transparent microemulsions, with a droplet size of <50 nm [11], while SNEDDS produce transparent dispersions of oil and water stabilized by surfactants, with droplet sizes between 20 and 250 nm and kinetically but not thermodynamically stable systems [29]. These two systems are the most famous colloidal dispersions within lipid-based systems but physicochemically different. Structures and properties of nanoemulsion can be changed on long-term storage but not for microemulsions at same temperature, pressure and composition. The formation of SMEDDS is spontaneous, and SNEDDS need high-energy methods for their fabrication, but both systems need some external energy to overcome kinetic energy barriers and support mass transport. In comparison, SNEDDS need lesser surfactant-to-oil ratio than SMEDDS. The preparation of SNEDDS involve specific mixing order in which surfactant must be mixed first with oil phase, whereas SMEDDS do not need any specific mixing order for their preparation. Ternary phase diagrams are required to have a suitable selection of both systems which should be coherent with different phases involved in preparation.

An important best-known example is Sandimmune Neoral® which was introduced in 1994 became the turning point for development of SMEDDS in oral lipid-based formulations of PWSD [30]. This formulation contains Cremophor RH40 (polyoxyl hydrogenated castor oil), corn oil glycerides, propylene glycol and ethanol, which emulsifies spontaneously into a microemulsion with a particle size smaller than 100 nm. This new formulation (Sandimmune Neoral®) resulted in a twofold increase in the bioavailability compared to the earlier product Sandimmune® [31]. Recent years, SMEDDS and SNEDDS have gained lots of interest as potential drug delivery vehicles largely due to their clarity, simplicity of preparation, thermodynamic stability and their abilities to be filtered and to incorporate a wide range of drugs of varying lipophilicity.

4.1.1. SMEDDS/SNEDDS within lipid formulation classification systems

By considering several factors in mind, Pouton [20, 32] introduced a lipid formulation classification system (LFCS) into four Types (I–IV) which differentiate lipid-based formulations from one to another that is being used as a framework to categorize nanoformulations. These four Types of formulations were classified on the basis of formulation compositions, their aqueous dispersibility and the potential effects of lipid digestion and possible drug precipitation from lipids. Among the LFCS, Type III systems are the most attractive formulations as they produce microemulsions/nanoemulsions (SMEDDS and SNEDDS) of lipid-surfactant mixtures with particle sizes in the range of 0–250 nm upon dispersion. The microemulsions can be used for many other drug delivery/application systems, such as topical, intra venous, trans-dermal, etc. There are several marketed products available which were developed as Type III formulations since the drugs may be absorbed from the microemulsions and or nanoemulsions without the digestion of lipids and/or surfactants present. Type III systems further divided into subtype IIIA and IIIB according to the hydrophilic content of the SMEDDS and SNEDDS. Type IV systems are efficient formulations as they also produce SMEDDS and/or SNEDDS and have high drug loading ability but may loss solvent capacity upon dilution with aqueous media.

4.2. Solidification of SMEDDS/SNEDDS

The excipients commonly used in designing SNEDDS are liquid at room temperature, and their compatibility with semi-solid and solid dosage forms allows encapsulating into soft/hard gelatin capsules for oral delivery. This could be a great challenge as the interaction between liquid formulation and capsule shell may result in either brittleness or softness of the shell [33]. In addition, the stability of liquid formulations could be another major issue (e.g., leaching and rancidity) since some drugs might suffer significant chemical instability in both aqueous and oily formulations. Apart from that, manufacturing liquid-filled soft gelatin capsules is a slow process and requires specialized equipment, having risk of formulation components migrating into capsule shell [23].

Therefore, to address this limitation, incorporation of liquid lipid formulations into a solid dosage form is convincing and desirable. Liquid lipid formulations could be transformed into acceptable free flowing fine powder by loading the formulation on a suitable solid carrier as solid SNEDDS [34, 35]. Only few studies have attempted to investigate the conversion of such formulations into free flowing powders by adsorption using various inorganic high surface area materials (i.e., neusilin, syloid, aeroperal and aerosol) that are amenable to encapsulation or tableting [36, 37]. On the other hand, the final powder preparation should have acceptable flow properties to achieve the best content uniformity and weight variation. The current interest in solidification technique by both the industry and academia is raised enormously due to the attractive properties including independence of gastric transit, flexibility in dose dividing, decrease in intra- and inter-subject variability, highest safety profile and physical/chemical stability improvement.

5. Equilibrium solubility of diluted nanoformulations

For lipid nanoformulations, drug solubility determines the maximum drug loading capacity (single unit dose) and is increased when the drug is highly lipid soluble or when the formulation contains high proportions of surfactant or cosolvent. The solubilization capacity of the nanoformulations (SNEDDS) is likely to decrease when excipients are dispersed and digested

http://dx.doi.org/10.5772/65710

in the GI tract. As a result, the drug concentrations in the GI fluids are elevated from the equilibrium solubility and could cause extreme precipitation.

To predict the likely fate of the drug on dispersion effectively, one should investigate its solubility in the formulations during aqueous dilution. The solubility of PWSDs within the diluted nanoformulations can be determined using a shake-flask method to observe how the drug solubility is changed as water is incorporated into the system. The samples are prepared by adding an excess amount of drug to the formulation, which is then shaken and thoroughly mixed with a vortex mixer. The samples are incubated in a dry heat incubator at 37°C for 7 days and centrifuged to separate excess solid drug from the dissolved drug. An aliquot of the supernatant is weighed and diluted in an appropriate solvent. The dissolved drug concentration can be analyzed by UV-vis spectrophotometer.

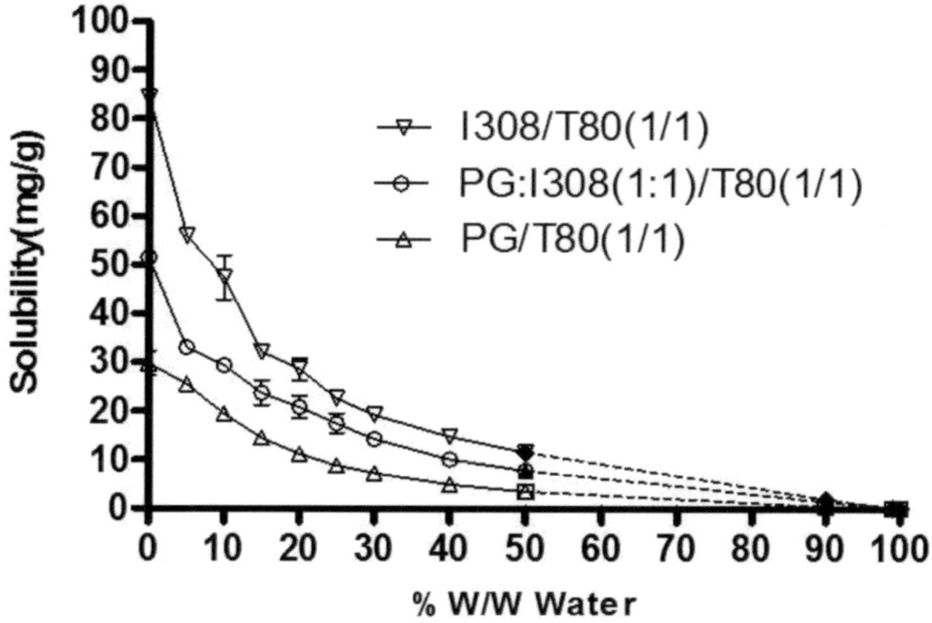

Figure 2. Effect of aqueous dilution on solubility of fenofibrate in nanoformulations representing LFCS Types IIIB and IV systems. Data are presented as mean ± SD (n = 3).

Figure 2 shows the fenofibrate solubility in nanoformulations (SMEDDS/SNEDDS) of LFCS Type IIIB and IV systems which was studied over 10–100 dilution with water. The results suggest how fenofibrate solubility decreased markedly, with several Type IIIB and IV nanoformulations, as the formulation was diluted with water [12]. After adding only 10% w/w water to the anhydrous formulation (drug dissolved at 80% of its equilibrium solubility), the one-third drug solubility had dropped down from the initial solubility of the formulation. The data predict that if fenofibrate was dissolved at its equilibrium solubility in the anhydrous formulations, its solubility would be exceeded in all cases when the formulation is diluted 1 in 10 or 1 in 100.

6. Drug release and the justification of dispersion test for nanoformulations

In vitro release studies assess the ability of lipid-based nanoformulations to disperse into various types of media and to evaluate whether the drug partitions from the vehicle into the aqueous medium. It can estimate how much drug will be in solution before absorption thus predicts the fate of the drug *in vivo*. A range of biorelevant dissolution test media and experimental methodologies has been developed by Dressman's group that have established application in drug release studies from lipid-based oral formulations [38, 39].

Technically, it is difficult to characterize drug release from emulsions *in vitro*, particularly under sink condition. Since solubility of the drug in sink phase may be poor, large volumes of aqueous content may be needed to maintain the sink conditions. It is hard to separate the oil droplets due to their smaller size from the dissolved or released drug in the sink solution levy. In a previous study, our group has conducted an *in vitro* dissolution of anti-histaminic drug, cinnarizine (CN, week base) from various SNEDDS systems and commercial product Stugeron® tablet [4]. Dissolution was carried out in simulated gastric fluid (SGF, pH 1.2) for first 2 h and subsequently shifted into simulated intestinal fluid (SIF, pH 6.8) for another 2 h.

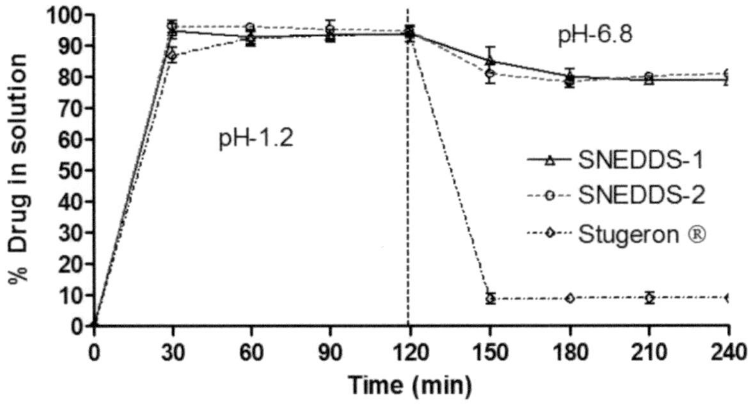

Figure 3. Dissolution profiles of cinnarizine SNEDDS 1 [MCT/MCDM/T85 (25/25/50)], SNEDDS 2 [MCT/MCM/T85 (25/25/50)] and Stugeron® tablets. Data are expressed as mean ± S.E, n = 3. **Abbreviations: MCT—medium-chain triglycerides (M810); MCDM—mixture of medium-chain di- and monoglycerides (I988); MCM—medium-chain monoglycerides (I308); T85—Tween 85.

In SGF, all the SNEDDS showed superior dissolution profiles with respect to Stugeron® tablet (**Figure 3**). At 15 min, Stugeron® tablet managed to release only 66.5% drug in solution where the optimal formulations were able to release 84–95% drug in solution. This indicates the ability of these formulations to provide more efficient and rapid release of CN with respect to the marketed tablet. Upon shifting from SGF to SIF, Stugeron® showed significant precipitation (87–92% precipitated), while the SNEDDS were able to hold high amount of CN (78–93%) in solution (**Figure 3**). This finding suggests the immense need for developing a SNEDDS that could enhance the drug dissolution profile and resist the sharp pH-dependent changes particularly for week bases.

A standard USP dissolution apparatus is suitable for the establishment of a dispersion test, but emphasis should be on precipitation rather than dissolution [4]. This is why, dynamic dispersion test is highly considered for the prediction of whether precipitation is likely to occur prior to digestion. In the dispersion study, samples are removed from the dispersion vessel at various intervals for at least 24 h and analyzed to determine the likelihood of precipitation during GI transit. Dispersion testing is vital for LFCS Types III and IV formulations (produce SNEDDS), which may loss solvent capacity on dispersion due to migration of water soluble components into the bulk aqueous phase. Care is needed in the design of lipid-based nanoformulations to ensure that the precipitation of the drug is minimized.

7. Mechanism of drug supersaturation: role of SMEDDS/SNEDDS

When the lipid nanoformulations approach to the high volume of gastric fluid, it is dispersed rapidly and reduces solubilization capacity of the drug due to the high content of surfactant/water soluble cosolvent, thus potentially generates supersaturation. Even though supersaturation in the stomach is not desirable as most of the drugs are absorbed in the small intestine, it poses threat for drug precipitation before the drug enters to small intestine. Therefore, SMEDDS/SNEDDS should be designed to minimize supersaturation in the stomach or at least to maintain a period sufficient to allow gastric emptying prior to drug precipitation.

Correlations between the investigations of the equilibrium solubility of the drug in the aqueous diluted formulation (10–99% diluted) and corresponding dynamic dispersion tests could help to predict whether precipitation is likely to take place, and whether it would affect bioavailability [12]. The imbalance between high initial solubilized drug concentrations and lower equilibrium drug solubilities during lipid dispersion and digestion *in vivo* does not immediately result in precipitation but stimulates drug supersaturation. This supersaturation is more likely to occur in the formulations that contain high proportions of water soluble surfactants or cosolvent. In some cases, during the process of lipid (or surfactant) digestion where hydrolysis occurs to form more polar post digestion products also stimulates changes to colloidal structure, thus lead to changes in drug solubility and may facilitate drug precipitation.

This is why, SNEDDS must contain drugs less than equilibrium solubility (approximately 50–90% of the equilibrium solubility) to avoid any precipitation. In recent studies, precipitation inhibitors have been introduced in supersaturated SNEDDS to overcome the risk of precipitations [40]. Supersaturated SNEDDS inhibit and minimize the nucleation process and subsequent drug precipitation in GIT by achieving and then sustaining the metastable supersaturated state. The commonly used water soluble precipitation inhibitors are PVP, HPMC, NaCMC and MC polymers [41].

7.1. The risk of drug precipitation from nanoformulations

Triglycerides alone (LFCS Type I) are poor solvents for most of the hydrophobic drugs but suitable for highly lipophilic compounds. If lipid-based formulations contain mixed glycerides, polar oils, surfactants and/or cosolvents (LFCS Type II and III), it is likely to improve the solvent capacity of the formulation. Therefore, formulators are always preferred to add water soluble surfactants and cosolvents against pure oils, ultimately sometimes resulting in the complete exclusion of oily excipients to produce oil-free formulations (LFCS Type IV). However, the formulator must keep well balance between oils and surfactants/cosolvents in the formulation to avoid risk of drug precipitation on aqueous dispersion. Several studies showed that small changes in formulation compositions are not expected to cause large changes in drug solubility, but there could be a dramatic drop in solvent capacity upon aqueous dilution [4, 12, 42]. Dilution of a cosolvent implies a substantial loss of solvent capacity, while the loss of solvent capacity may not be suffered with the use of surfactant. This could be possible due to the linearity between solubilized drug to the number of micelles present and therefore to the surfactant concentration. Drugs which are more soluble in surfactant or cosolvent than pure oil are at high precipitation risk because solvent capacity of surfactant and cosolvent decreases upon dilution but not pure oil. Hence, increasing the solubility of a drug by including a cosolvent is generally a poor strategy than using a nonionic surfactant [11, 43]. **Figure 4** shows the extreme precipitation of an anticancer drug, paclitaxel using LFCS Types III and IV formulations.

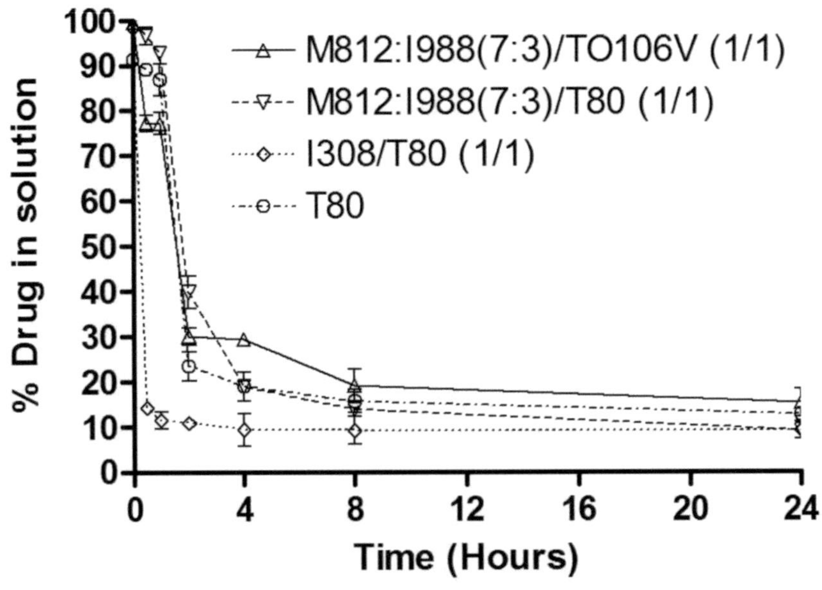

Figure 4. Percentage of the original dose of paclitaxel remaining in solution after 1:100 dilutions in the dispersion medium (paclitaxel was originally dissolved at 80% of the equilibrium solubility in the anhydrous mixture). One gram formulation was dispersed in 100 ml water, and then, the samples were withdrawn periodically over 24 h to examine the drug precipitations. Data are presented as mean ± SD (n = 3).

It is quite difficult to predict the fate of the PWSDs on dispersion of a typical LFCS Type IIIA lipid formulation. The hydrophilic surfactant used in Type IIIA systems is substantially separated from the oily components, forming a micellar solution in the continuous phase.

Hence, one might question: does this system lower the overall solvent capacity for the drug or not? However, this may depend on the log *P* of the drug, and to what extent the surfactant was contributing to its solubilization within the formulation. At present, there are no established techniques available to help formulators assessing the risk of precipitation. It is worth mentioning that in some cases, Type III formulations can take several days to reach equilibrium and the drug remains in a supersaturated state for up to 24 h time [12]. It could be argued that such formulations are not likely to cause precipitation in the gut before the drug is absorbed, and possibly the supersaturation acts as an absorption enhancer by increasing the thermodynamic stability of the drug [44].

8. Lipid digestion and drug absorption: mechanism

8.1. Lipid metabolism

Following ingestion of a lipid-based dosage form (capsule/tablet), the formulation is initially dispersed in the stomach where the digestion of exogenous dietary lipid is started by the action of gastric lipase on the lipid-water interface. Gastric lipase releases about 15% of free fatty acids from lipids [45]. Within the small intestine, pancreatic lipase together with its co-lipase completes the breakdown of dietary glycerides to diglyceride, monoglyceride and fatty acid. The presence of exogenous lipids in the small intestine also stimulates secretion of endogenous biliary lipids including bile salt, phospholipid and cholesterol from the gallbladder [45]. In the presence of elevated bile salts concentrations, lipid digestion products are subsequently incorporated into a series of colloidal structures including multilamellar/unilamellar vesicles, bile salt phospholipid mixed micelles and micelles [46]. Together these species significantly expand the solubilization capacity of the small intestine for both lipid digestion products and drugs, and this can be studied relatively easily as a preformulation exercise.

8.2. Drug absorption

Sufficient aqueous solubility along with good intestinal permeability is crucial for adequate drug absorption, ultimately leading to sufficient bioavailability. On the other hand, PWSDs are associated with poor and variable absorption and often affected by the various food intakes. Several studies have already documented lipid-based nanoformulations, particularly SNEDDS, as an absorption enhancer for PWSDs when administered orally [4, 47]. Possible mechanisms for improving drug absorption include: (i) an increase in the membrane fluidity facilitating transcellular absorption, (ii) larger surface area provided by the fine emulsion droplets, hydrolysis and formation of mixed micelles, (iii) paracellular transport by opening tight junction mainly for ionized drugs or hydrophilic macromolecules, (iv) inhibition of P-gp and/or CYP450 to increase intracellular concentration and residence time, and (v) stimulation of lipoprotein/chylomicron production. The natural process of digestion offers the possibility that very lipophilic drugs could be taken up into the lymphatic system by partitioning into chylomicrons in the mesentery. This is expected to be a mechanism of absorption for drugs with log *P* values >6.0 and has been demonstrated to be crucial in a past study for the absorption of the antimalarial compound halofantrine [48, 49].

The mixed micelles substantially transport digestion products across the unstirred water layer and reach the vicinity of the aqueous-microvillus interface to allow for lipid absorption through the mucosal cells. However, it is possible that digestion of a lipid formulation could reduce the solubility of the drug in the gut lumen, which would result in the precipitation of the drug and a decrease in the absorption rate. Therefore, more investigation on *in vitro* lipolysis is needed to clearly understand drug precipitation during digestion for better absorption.

9. *In vitro* digestion (lipolysis): significance

The fate of the lipid carrier in the GI tract is essentially important for the absorption of the incorporated drug and therefore has to be closely analyzed. It is evident that the solvent capacity of the formulation can be lost on digestion, leading to drug precipitation [26, 50]. However, the investigation of the lipolysis by *in vivo* experiments is complex, costly and time-consuming. Thus, the *in vitro* model simulating the enzymatic degradation of lipid-based formulations is highly significant as an alternative method of monitoring the digestion process in the simulated gastrointestinal media under fed and fasted conditions.

Lipolysis can be carried out as an *in vitro* test using a pH-stat titration unit to maintain pH and using the lipase/co-lipase content of porcine pancreatin to serve as model for human pancreatic juice. Bile salt lecithin-mixed micelles are used in the reaction mixture to provide a sink for solubilization of degradation products. Composition of mixture that used in the *in vitro* lipolysis studies is provided in **Table 2**.

Substance of the mixture for 10 ml aqueous media		
Lipid 250 mg		
Pancreatic lipase 1 ml (800 TBU/ml)		
Lipolysis buffer 9 ml		
Composition of the lipolysis buffer	**Concentration (fed state)**	**Concentration (fasted state)**
Bile salt (BS, mM)	20	5
Phospholipid (PL, mM)	5	1.25
Trizma maleate (mM)	0.5	0.5
Ca^+ (mM)	0.05	0.05
Na^+ (mM)	1.5	1.5

Table 2. Composition of mixture for *in vitro* lipolysis experiments. *Adapted with permission from Ref. [51].

Lipolysis is allowed to proceed for a fixed time (30–60 min), the reaction is then subjected to high-speed ultracentrifugation, and further drug analysis in the various phases allows predicting whether the drug will remain solubilized in the intestinal lumen after digestion of the formulation. However, if the drug is partially precipitated, then drug will be found in the pellet, which may be still in solution. The rate and extent of lipolysis can be quantified by the data generated from the pH-stat. This technique was recently applied in LFCS Types I–IV formulations to predict the effect of formulation on the fate of a number of drug compounds and assumed that surfactants are subjected to digestion, probably for SMEDDS and SNEDDS, where water soluble surfactants are used predominantly. Lipolysis experiments may play a vital role in the near future for establishing strong methods for *in vitro in vivo* correlations (*IVIVCs*).

10. *In vitro in vivo* correlation (*IVIVC*) for lipid nanoformulations

The *IVIVCs* play a major role in drug development, particularly on the optimization of suitable formulations which is time-consuming and a highly expensive process. Formulation optimization requires modifications in composition, equipment, manufacturing process and batch sizes. If such changes applied to the formulation, the *in vivo* bioequivalence studies in human are necessary to be conducted to confirm the similarity of the new formulation. This process will increase the load of carrying out a number of bioequivalence studies and therefore will increase the cost of process optimization and marketing of the new formulation.

To overcome these issues, it is necessary to develop *in vitro* tests that can imitate the bioavailability data. The *IVIVC* can be used in the development of new pharmaceuticals to decrease the number of human trials during the formulation development and to support biowaivers.

In the beginning of 1980s, the *IVIVC* theory was established based on many published research studies, which can be used as a prediction tool for correlating *in vitro* and *in vivo* data. The *IVIVC* is usually used in the development stages of pharmaceuticals to enhance the formulation and dosage optimization with fewer trials in human [51–56] or additional bioavailability studies. The FDA defines *IVIVC* as "a predictive mathematical model describing the relationship between an *in vitro* property of a dosage form (usually the rate or extent of drug dissolution or release) and a relevant *in vivo* response (e.g., plasma drug concentration or amount of drug absorbed)." For drugs that are administered orally, dissolution and intestinal permeation are considered as the rate-limiting steps for the absorption. Therefore, if an excellent correlation exists between *in vitro* dissolution test and a bioavailability parameter, then controlling the dissolution profile will permit the evaluation of bioavailability [57–59].

There are several tools which can be used to establish *IVIVC*. The *in vitro* drug release studies of the formulations can be performed using dissolution, dynamic dispersion and digestion tests, whereas the *in vivo* pharmacokinetic studies can be performed on various animal models. However, there are only a limited number of *IVIVC* studies so far have been conducted using lipid formulations. To obtain more robust *in vitro* and *in vivo* relationship, a large number of model compounds should be explored along with more human clinical data sets and complete characterizations of *in vitro* and *in vivo* solubilization of PWSDs formulated in lipid vehicles.

11. Conclusion

For many drugs with poor aqueous solubility, the technique of developing SMEDDS/SNEDDS provides a powerful and effective solution to improve their solubility in the aqueous contents of the GI tract that is the main obstacle for such drugs. The most critical step in designing the nanoformulations of lipid-based systems for PWSDs is the selection of the most suitable oil, surfactant and/or cosolvent for a particular drug with certain physicochemical properties. So, the formulators must keep a balance and make compatibility between the factors of different formulations such as self-emulsification efficiency, drug loading capacity, droplet size distribution, *in vitro* dispersion/release profile in acidic and basic media and *in vitro* digestion by using fed and fasted state. In summary, SMEDDS/SNEDDS provide a robust formulation approach to enhance GI solubilization and to promote drug absorption after oral administration. If there is a successful *IVIVC* made for lipid nanoformulations, confidence in the development of the pharmaceutical product and its quality are likely to improve, and the drug development time may be shortened.

Author details

Mohsin Kazi

Address all correspondence to: mkazi@ksu.edu.sa

Department of Pharmaceutics, College of Pharmacy, King Saud University, Riyadh, Kingdom of Saudi Arabia

References

[1] Lei, Y., et al., Solid self-nanoemulsifying cyclosporin A pellets prepared by fluid-bed coating: preparation, characterization and *in vitro* redispersibility. Int. J. Nanomed., 2011. 6: p. 795–805.

[2] Kommuru, T.R., et al., Self-emulsifying drug delivery systems (SEDDS) of coenzyme Q10: formulation development and bioavailability assessment. Int. J. Pharm., 2001. 212(2): p. 233–246.

[3] Mohsin, K., A.A. Shahba, and F.K. Alanazi, Lipid based self emulsifying formulations for poorly water soluble drugs-an excellent opportunity. Indian J. Pharm. Educ. Res., 2012. 46(2): p. 88–96.

[4] Shahba, A.A., K. Mohsin, and F.K. Alanazi, Novel self-nanoemulsifying drug delivery systems (SNEDDS) for oral delivery of cinnarizine: design, optimization, and *in-vitro* assessment. AAPS PharmSciTech, 2012. 13(3): p. 967–977.

[5] Mueller, E.A., et al., Improved dose linearity of cyclosporine pharmacokinetics from a microemulsion formulation. Pharm. Res., 1994. 11(2): p. 301–304.

[6] Date, A.A., et al., Self-nanoemulsifying drug delivery systems: formulation insights, applications and advances. Nanomedicine (Lond), 2010. 5(10): p. 1595–1616.

[7] Date, A.A. and M.S. Nagarsenker, Design and evaluation of self-nanoemulsifying drug delivery systems (SNEDDS) for cefpodoxime proxetil. Int. J. Pharm., 2007. 329(1–2): p. 166–172.

[8] Charman, S.A., et al., Self-emulsifying drug delivery systems: formulation and biopharmaceutic evaluation of an investigational lipophilic compound. Pharm. Res., 1992. 9(1): p. 87–93.

[9] Charman, W.N., et al., Effect of food and a monoglyceride emulsion formulation on danazol bioavailability. J. Clin. Pharmacol., 1993. 33(4): p. 381–386.

[10] Gursoy, R.N. and S. Benita, Self-emulsifying drug delivery systems (SEDDS) for improved oral delivery of lipophilic drugs. Biomed. Pharmacother., 2004. 58(3): p. 173–182.

[11] Pouton, C.W., Formulation of poorly water-soluble drugs for oral administration: physicochemical and physiological issues and the lipid formulation classification system. Eur. J. Pharm. Sci., 2006. 29(3–4): p. 278–287.

[12] Mohsin, K., M.A. Long, and C.W. Pouton, Design of lipid-based formulations for oral administration of poorly water-soluble drugs: precipitation of drug after dispersion of formulations in aqueous solution. J. Pharm. Sci., 2009. 98(10): p. 3582–3595.

[13] Duro, R., et al., Interfacial adsorption of polymers and surfactants: implications for the properties of disperse systems of pharmaceutical interest. Drug Dev. Ind. Pharm., 1999. 25(7): p. 817–829.

[14] Floyd, A.G., Top ten considerations in the development of parenteral emulsions. Pharm. Sci. Technol. Today, 1999. 4(2): p. 134–143.

[15] Pouton, C.W., Effects of the inclusion of a model drug on the performance of self emulsifying formulations. J. Pharm. Pharmacol., 1984. 36: p. 51.

[16] Pouton, C.W., Self emulsifying drug delivery systems: assessment of the efficiency of emulsification. Int. J. Pharm., 1985. 27: p. 335–348.

[17] Tarr, B.D. and S.H. Yalkowsky, Enhanced intestinal absorption of cyclosporine in rats through the reduction of emulsion droplet size. Pharm. Res., 1989. 6(1): p. 40–43.

[18] Humberstone, A.J. and W.N. Charman, Lipid based vehicles for the oral delivery of poorly water soluble drugs. Adv. Drug Deliv. Rev., 1997. 25(1): p. 103–128.

[19] Jannin, V., J. Musakhanian, and D. Marchaud, Approaches for the development of solid and semi-solid lipid-based formulations. Adv. Drug Deliv. Rev., 2008. 60(6): p. 734–746.

[20] Pouton, C. and C. Porter, Formulation of lipid-based delivery systems for oral administration: materials, methods and strategies. Adv. Drug Deliv. Rev., 2008. 60(6): p. 625–637.

[21] Mohsin, K., et al., Development of self-nanoemulsifying drug delivery systems for the enhancement of solubility and oral bioavailability of fenofibrate, a poorly water-soluble drug. Int. J. Nanomed., 2016. 11: p. 2829–2838.

[22] Cerpnjak, K., et al., Lipid-based systems as a promising approach for enhancing the bioavailability of poorly water-soluble drugs. Acta Pharm., 2013. 63(4): p. 427–445.

[23] Perry, C.M. and S. Noble, Saquinavir soft-gel capsule formulation. A review of its use in patients with HIV infection. Drugs, 1998. 55(3): p. 461–486.

[24] Hoffmann-La-Roche, *Fortovase (saquinavir) Soft Gelatin Capsules. Product Information.* (CAS registry number: 127779-20-8), 2003; http://www.medicines.org.au/files/ropforto.pdf

[25] Martin-Facklam, M., et al., Dose-dependent increase of saquinavir bioavailability by the pharmaceutic aid cremophor EL. Br. J. Clin. Pharmacol., 2002. 53(6): p. 576–581.

[26] Porter, C.J. and W.N. Charman, *In vitro* assessment of oral lipid based formulations. Adv. Drug Deliv. Rev., 2001. 50(Suppl 1): p. S127–S147.

[27] Talegaonkar, S., et al., Microemulsions: a novel approach to enhanced drug delivery. Recent Pat. Drug Deliv. Formul., 2008. 2(3): p. 238–257.

[28] Singh, B., et al., Self-emulsifying drug delivery systems (SEDDS): formulation development, characterization, and applications. Crit. Rev. Ther. Drug Carrier Syst., 2009. 26(5): p. 427–521.

[29] Cherniakov, I., A.J. Domb, and A. Hoffman, Self-nano-emulsifying drug delivery systems: an update of the biopharmaceutical aspects. Expert Opin. Drug Deliv., 2015. 12(7): p. 1121–1133.

[30] Klyashchitsky, B.A. and A.J. Owen, Drug delivery systems for cyclosporine: achievements and complications. J. Drug Target, 1998. 5(6): p. 443–458.

[31] Mueller, E.A., et al., Influence of a fat-rich meal on the pharmacokinetics of a new oral formulation of cyclosporine in a crossover comparison with the market formulation. Pharm. Res., 1994. 11(1): p. 151–155.

[32] Pouton, C.W., Lipid formulations for oral administration of drugs: non-emulsifying, self-emulsifying and 'self-microemulsifying' drug delivery systems. Eur. J. Pharm. Sci., 2000. 11(Suppl 2): p. S93–S98.

[33] Nazzal, S. and M. Khan, Controlled release of a self-emulsifying formulation from a tablet dosage form: stability assessment and optimization of some processing parameters. Int. J. Pharm., 2006. 315(1–2): p. 110–121.

[34] Tang, B., G. Cheng, J-C. Gu, and C-H. Xu, Development of solid self-emulsifying drug delivery systems: preparation techniques and dosage forms. Drug Discov. Today, 2008. 13: p. 606–612.

[35] Katteboina, S., P. Chandrasekhar, and S. Balaji, Approaches for the development of solid self-emulsifying drug delivery systems and dosage forms. Asian J. Pharm. Sci., 2009. 4: p. 240–253.

[36] Agarwal, V., A. Siddiqui, H. Ali, and S. Nazzal, Dissolution and powder flow characterization of solid self-emulsified drug delivery system (SEDDS). Int. J. Pharm., 2009. 366: p. 44–52.

[37] Shazly, G. and K. Mohsin, Dissolution improvement of solid self-emulsifying drug delivery systems of fenofibrate using an inorganic high surface adsorption material. Acta Pharm., 2015. 65(1): p. 29–42.

[38] Dressman, J.B. and Klein, S., eds. Development of dissolution tests on the basis of gastrointestinal physiology. Pharmaceutical Dissolution Testing, eds. Dressman, J., and Krämer, J., 2005, Taylor and Francis: NY, USA. pp. 193–227.

[39] Dressman, J.B., Alsenz, J., Schamp, K., and Beltz, K., eds. Characterizing release from lipid-based formulations. Oral Lipid-based Formulations: Enhancing the Bioavailability of Poorly Water-soluble Drugs, eds. Hauss, DJ., 2007, Informa Healthcare, Inc.: NY, USA. pp. 242–245.

[40] Thomas, N., K. Richter, T.B. Pedersen, R. Holm, A. Müllertz, and T. Rades, *In vitro* lipolysis data does not adequately predict the *in vivo* performance of lipid-based drug delivery systems containing fenofibrate. AAPS J., 2014. 16(3): p. 539–549.

[41] Gao, P., et al., Enhanced oral bioavailability of a poorly water soluble drug PNU-91325 by supersaturatable formulations. Drug Dev. Ind. Pharm., 2004. 30(2): p. 221–229.

[42] Mohsin, K. and F. Alanazi, The fate of paclitaxel during *in vitro* dispersion testing of different lipid-based formulations. J. Drug Deliv. Sci. Technol., 2012. 22(2): p. 197–204.

[43] Devraj, R., et al., *In vitro* assessment of drug-free and fenofibrate-containing lipid formulations using dispersion and digestion testing gives detailed insights into the likely fate of formulations in the intestine. Eur. J. Pharm. Sci., 2013. 49(4): p. 748–760.

[44] Gao, P., B.D. Rush, W.P. Pfund, T. Huang, J.M. Bauer, W. Morozowich, M.S. Kuo, and M.J. Hageman, Development of a supersaturable SEDDS (S-SEDDS) formulation of paclitaxel with improved oral bioavailability. J. Pharm. Sci., 2003. 92: p. 2386–2398.

[45] Porter, C.J., N.L. Trevaskis, and W.N. Charman, Lipids and lipid-based formulations: optimizing the oral delivery of lipophilic drugs. Nat. Rev. Drug Discov., 2007. 6(3): p. 231–248.

[46] Kossena, G.A., et al., Influence of the intermediate digestion phases of common formulation lipids on the absorption of a poorly water-soluble drug. J. Pharm. Sci., 2005. 94(3): p. 481–492.

[47] Stegemann, S., et al., Self-emulsifying drug delivery systems facing the bioavailability challenge in drug delivery. Pharm. Ind., 2009. 71(8): p. 1409–1416.

[48] Humberstone, A.J., C.J. Porter, and W.N. Charman, A physicochemical basis for the effect of food on the absolute oral bioavailability of halofantrine. J. Pharm. Sci., 1996. 85(5): p. 525–529.

[49] Boyd, M., et al., A stepwise surgical procedure to investigate the lymphatic transport of lipid-based oral drug formulations: cannulation of the mesenteric and thoracic lymph ducts within the rat. J. Pharmacol. Toxicol Methods, 2004. 49(2): p. 115–120.

[50] Pouton, C.W. and C.J. Porter, Formulation of lipid-based delivery systems for oral administration: materials, methods and strategies. Adv. Drug Deliv. Rev., 2008. 60(6): p. 625–637.

[51] Uppoor, V.R., Regulatory perspectives on *in vitro* (dissolution)/*in vivo* (bioavailability) correlations. J. Control. Release, 2001. 72(1–3): p. 127–132.

[52] Ghosh, P., M. Milewski, and K. Paudel, *In vitro/in vivo* correlations in transdermal product development. Ther. Deliv., 2015. 6(9): p. 1117–1124.

[53] Anand, O., et al., Dissolution testing for generic drugs: an FDA perspective. AAPS J., 2011. 13(3): p. 328–335.

[54] FDA, Guidance for Industry: Dissolution Testing of Immediate Release Solid Oral Dosage Forms, Food and Drug Administration, Rockville, 1997.

[55] Committee, I.C.o.H.S. Pharmaceutical Development Q8; Draft Consensus Guideline, Released for Consultation at Step 2 of the ICH Process; International Conference on Harmonisation of Technical Requirements for Registration of Pharmaceuticals for Human Use in International Conference on Harmonisation. 2004.

[56] European Agency for the Evaluation of Medicinal Products, H.M.E.U., Committee for Proprietary Medicinal Products, CPMP/QWP/155/96, *Note for Guidance on Development Pharmaceutics,* H.M.E.U. European Agency for the Evaluation of Medicinal Products, Committee for Proprietary Medicinal Products, CPMP/QWP/155/96, Editor 1998: London, UK.

[57] Hwang, S.S., W. Bayne, and F. Theeuwes, *In vivo* evaluation of controlled-release products. J. Pharm. Sci., 1993. 82(11): p. 1145–1150.

[58] Abd-Elbary, A., M.I. Tadros, and A.A. Alaa-Eldin, Development and *in vitro/in vivo* evaluation of etodolac controlled porosity osmotic pump tablets. AAPS PharmSciTech, 2011. 12(2): p. 485–495.

[59] Benet, L.Z., Pharmacokinetics of sustained-release etodolac. Rheumatol. Int., 1993. 13(Suppl 2): p. S3–S5.

Chapter 4

Hybrid Nano-carriers for Potential Drug Delivery

Asadullah Madni, Nayab Tahir, Mubashar Rehman,
Ahmed Raza, Muhammad Ahmad Mahmood,
Muhammad Imran Khan and
Prince Muhammad Kashif

Additional information is available at the end of the chapter

http://dx.doi.org/10.5772/66466

Abstract

Nanocarriers have provided the versatile platform for the delivery of various therapeutic and diagnostic agents. Liposome, niosomes, polymeric and solid lipid nanoparticles are the most promising nanocarriers that have been entered in the clinical trials and become commercially available. However, each system has been associated with some problems that can be minimized by using the combinatorial approach of hybrid nanocarriers. These hybrid systems combine the benefits of different structural components to synergize the outcome of the therapy. In this chapter, the different types of hybrid nanocarriers have been described with particular emphasis on the brief rationale for the development of these hybrid nanocarriers along with different fabrication approaches with greater emphasize on the lipid polymer hybrid nanoparticles. A brief description factors governing the optimized response characteristics and their potential application of these hybrid nanoparticles are also presented.

Keywords: core shell hybrid nanoparticles, drug delivery, hybrid nanoparticles, nanoflowers

1. Introduction

In the recent decades, pharmaceutical nanotechnology has opened a new era for the research in the design and characterization of drug delivery systems (DDS) and biotechnological products. A variety of novel drug delivery systems and strategies emerged for diagnostic and therapeutic applications that explored the different structural components, fabrication methods and mechanisms of drug delivery and targeting [1]. These DDS emphasized on the use of multiple nanomaterials and therapeutic moieties that renovate the current pharmaceutical industry and biomedical sciences toward the better drug therapy [2]. These nanosized particles were utilized for the delivery of various molecules including different drugs, proteins, nucleic acid and other diagnostic agents. Some of these compounds may be encapsulated inside while others were adsorbed on the surface of these nanoparticles. These nanocarriers can amend the pharmacokinetics and pharmacodynamics of drug by enhancing the solubility, permeability and bioavailability in multiple ways. The availability of the encapsulated compound depends upon the nature of formulation components and the other external stimuli which enable the controlled as well as targeted delivery of these encapsulated compounds within the cellular microenvironment [3]. All these parameters ultimately achieve the higher concentration of the encapsulated drug that efficiently reaches the potential target site without affecting the normal tissues. These nanocarriers also aid to implement the concept of rational therapeutics by providing the tunable drug delivery systems based on the patient therapeutic demands.

Despite of excellent in-vitro performance, some drugs demonstrate poor in-vivo results because of low aqueous solubility, poor membrane penetrability, rapid clearance by the reticuloendothelial system, complex pathophysiological states of the disease and uncertain plasma levels leading to drug toxicity, thus, requiring such drug delivery systems that overcome these problems [4]. Latest developments in the material sciences, polymer engineering and nanotechnology have enabled multidisciplinary research to formulate and evaluate different novel drug delivery systems that claimed increased drug solubility, penetration and retention at the targeted site in the body [5].

Among the different nanoparticulate systems, nanoparticles of different composition and lipid based vesicular carriers (liposome, lipid nanocarriers, solid lipid nanoparticles and drug lipid conjugates) have been frequently employed for the medical applications. The nanoparticles may provide versatility in terms of composition. As, these include the polymeric nanocarriers, mesoporous nanoparticles, metal coated (gold, iron and silver), inorganic nanoparticles, quantum dots, carbon nanotubes, dendrimers and magnetic nanoparticles [6, 7]. Furthermore, all these systems were modified to mimic the desired therapeutic properties through different modification method and ligands such as (i) increase in the retention time and stability of the system, (ii) stimuli triggered release, (iii) targeted delivery of various agents and (iv) administration of dual modalities simultaneously [8, 9].

Liposomes and niosomes have been considered as most promising domains among the lipid vesicular carriers. Liposomes are defined as the lipid vesicles having the single or multiple layers of the lipid providing the encapsulation of different therapeutic moieties while niosomes have the same morphology but contain nonionic surfactants instead of phospholipids as major structural components. They provide the better biocompatibility profile, easy surface modification of the vesicles, versatility in the loading of hydrophobic and hydrophilic drugs and improved pharmacokinetic properties [10, 11]. However, drug leakage or fast release from the system, reproducibility, poor physical and chemical stability on storage, higher cost and scale up issues are the major drawbacks associated with the vesicular systems [12, 13].

Nanoparticles (polymeric, organic/inorganic, mesoporous silica, calcium carbonate and different metals, i.e., iron, silver and gold) established the second domain of the nanocarriers. These systems prove superiority in terms of smaller particle size, structural integrity, versatility in the polymeric materials, improved drug loading and release profile. They also provide the targeting capabilities in the case of magnetic iron oxide nanoparticles and better cellular interactions in case of organic and inorganic nanoparticles [14]. Similar to that of vesicular systems, these polymeric nanoparticles have some limitations in term of polymer toxicity, presence of toxic organic solvents, poor entrapment of hydrophilic drugs, polymer degradation and drug leakage before reaching the site of action [15].

The problems associated with the liposomes, polymeric nanoparticles and other carrier systems can be reduced by using a novel combinatorial approach of "hybrid nanoparticles" (HNPs) that utilizes the positive attributes of two different components. These hybrid nanoparticles (HNPs) exploit the benefits of both systems (lipid and polymer/organic and inorganic materials) and the release profile of drug is based on the erosion and degradation of the core material by hydrolysis with in turn determined by water permeation into the outer shell layer and composition of the polymer. The core materials may be protected by the application of multiple layers of the shell materials and the interface of these layer acts as a site for the functionalization of the carrier system for the dual modalities of treatment and diagnosis [16].

Similarly, core shell hybrid nanoparticles using different oils, metal oxides, organic and inorganic components also provide newer system that has multilayered structure having the inner core outer shell with a suitable lipid or oil at the interface to develop a core shell hybrid structure. Recently, use of green approach offer more facile and potentially successful system with the added advantage of solvent-free nanohybrids with greater efficiency.

Such novel system consists of three different structural components as follows:

(i) The inner most core made up of different polymers (poly-lactic-co-glycolic acid [PLGA], polycaprolactone [PCL] and chitosan), lipids (cationic, anionic, zwitterion and neutral phospholipids and nonionic surfactants), inorganic materials (silica, iron oxide) and organic materials (polysaccharides) that encapsulate the therapeutically active moiety.

(ii) The intermediate lipid layer that covers the polymeric/inorganic core and enhance the biocompatibility of that system. It also acts as barrier to minimize the drug leakage and control the rate of polymer/inorganic core degradation by controlling the water permeation into the core.

(iii) The outer most lipid or polymer-conjugate which act as a layer for functionalization of the system by making it target specific through the use of different ligands or increased its circulation and retention time by coating with the PEG. This layer may be modified with a suitably charged moiety to attach the antibodies, aptamer and other such molecules by electrostatic forces [17]. Different types of the hybrid nanocarriers having different morphology and different structural components **Figure 1**.

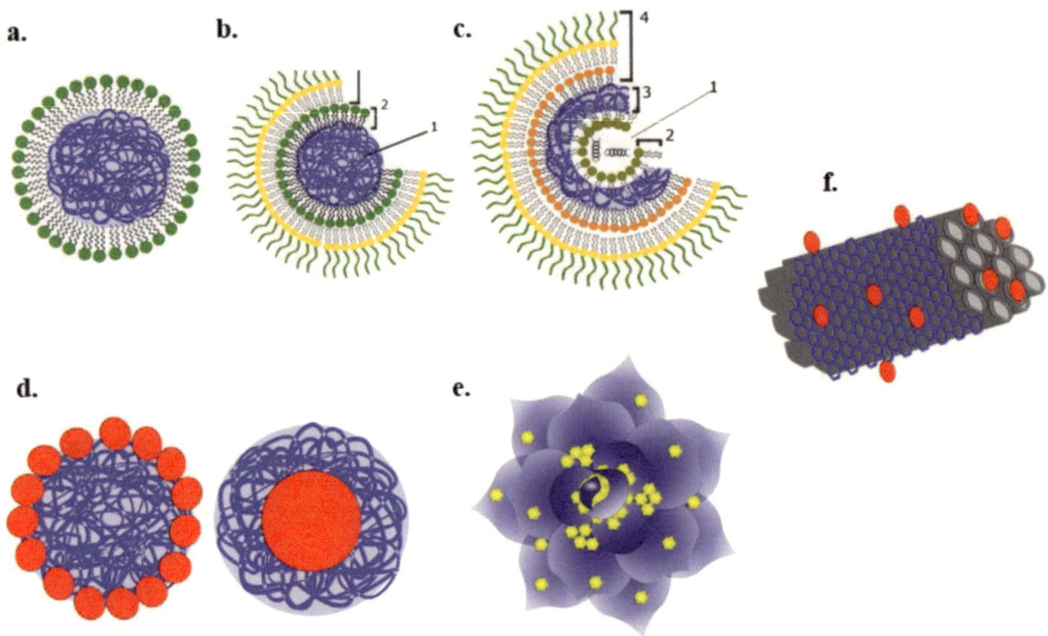

Figure 1. Structure of lipid-polymer hybrid nanoparticles; (a) polymer core-lipid shell hybrid, (b) 3 layers polymer-lipid hybrid nanoparticles consisting of polymeric core (1) and two lipid layers (2,3) shell, (c) 4 layers hollow core lipid-polymer hybrid, consisting of hollow core (1) covered by reverse surfactant layer (2), polymeric shell (3), and outer shells of two lipids (4). (d) organic core-inorganic shell and inorganic core-organic shell hybrid, (e) inorganic (metallic)-protein hybrid nanoflowers, and (f) graphene oxide coated mesoporous silica-inorganic hybrid nanoparticles.

In this chapter, the different types of hybrid nanocarriers have been described with particular emphasis on the brief rationale for the development of these hybrid nanocarriers along with different fabrication approaches with greater emphasize on the lipid polymer hybrid nanoparticles. A brief description factors governing the optimized response characteristics and their potential application of these hybrid nanoparticles are also presented.

2. Method of preparation

Different methods have been employed for the fabrication of hybrid nanocarriers depending upon their chemical composition and applications. The lipid-polymer hybrid, polymer-inorganic hybrid, metal (gold, silver or iron) polymer, silica (SiO_2) based hybrid nanosystems and hybrid polymeric nanocarriers have been most widely investigated [18]. Most of these hybrid carriers utilized two distinctive fabrication approaches. First, a two-step conventional approach process, in which the inner core and outer shell are prepared separately and then are coincubated for the formation of hybrid nanoparticle. The second approach is the single step, in which various state-of-the art techniques of the self-assembling are being incorporated. These processes are further modified with different chemical moieties to obtain versatile hybrid nanoparticles meeting specific need of therapy [19]. In the present chapter, we will focus on the two step conventional as well as single step formulation approaches along with recent innovations have been presented in order to prepare the hybrid nanocarriers with versatile characteristics.

2.1. Conventional two-step method

It was the first technique employed for the fabrication of hybrid nanocarriers. The inner core and outer shell components are prepared in two separate steps employing suitable polymers and chemicals and are then combined to form the hybrid nanoparticle [17]. The foremost type of core shell hybrid nanoparticles contained a core of the polymeric nanoparticles and an outer shell of preformed lipid component such as liposome or lipoparticles in appropriate ratios [20]. Further, the single or multilayered shell is prepared with other techniques such as sonication [21], extrusion or high pressure homogenization and vortexing [22]. The polymeric core is prepared by emulsification-solvent evaporation or solvent diffusion [23], desolvation [24], nanoprecipitation [25, 26], sonication [27] and high pressure homogenization [28] depending upon the hydrophobicity of the loading drugs, their applications [29] and the size of the core.

The single step method is applied when the core materials such as polymers, silica and organic substances are miscible with the drug payload and also are solubilized in the organic solvent [30, 31]. The double emulsification step is employed when the compound is immiscible with the organic solvents and does not form covalent linkage with the core material. As this method requires multiple steps for mixing of different components, relatively larger hybrid nanoparticles are produced [32]. Further, any of the suitable technique such as ultrasonication or extrusion by high pressure homogenization also reduces the particle size as the polymer solution is passed through the nozzle under high pressure. Furthermore, the freeze drying or cooling at normal temperature produced free flowing characteristic particles [33, 34]. Another recent innovation is the application of nanoprecipitation method for the preparation of polymeric core. The polymer is dissolve in the suitable solvent and then precipitated by using the nonsolvent component [26].

The formed polymeric core and lipid vesicles are mixed by vortexing, extrusion, film hydration and ultrasonication techniques in order to formulate the hybrid nanoparticles. The mixing processes provide the energy for the fusion or adsorption of the shell on the inner core material. Additionally, the electrostatic forces among these components also play their role for fabrication of hybrid nanoparticles [35]. It is worth mentioning here that mixing process must be carried out above the phase transition temperature of the lipid component. The formed hybrid nanoparticles are separated by the ultracentrifugation process [36, 37]. Different investigators such as Liang et al. [38] and Zhao et al. [39] prepared the hybrid nanoparticles and nanocells by the emulsification solvent evaporation technique employing the paclitaxel loaded polymeric nanoparticles as core and the PEG or folic acid conjugated octadecyl-quaternary lysine-modified chitosan and cholesterol as lipid shell [38, 39].

2.2. Modified two-step methods

The modifications to the conventional two step method such as spray drying and lithographic molding processes have also been employed for fabrication of hybrid nanoparticles [29]. The inner core is prepared by the spray drying which is dispersed in an appropriate solvent containing the lipid, polymer or any inorganic material. The spray dried lipid coated core shell hybrid nanoparticles were collected after the completion [17].

Freeze or spray dried inhalation hybrid nanoparticles of levofloxacin, ciprofloxacin and isoniazid coated with multiple layers of the lipids were prepared using double emulsion solvent evaporation technique. These hybrid nanoparticles showed better inhalation efficiency, emitted particle size and diameter compared to the conventional two step methods [37, 40]. Another investigations employed nanospray drying for fabrication of hybrid nanoparticles using polyglutamic acid, poly lysine nanoparticles coated with the lipid materials [41]. Recently, Keloglu et al. [42] employed jet spray drying technique for the fabrication of hybrid microfibers-nanoparticles having low density and greater strength using PLGA and poly lactic acid (PLA) [42].

A soft lithography particle molding technique was also utilized for the preparation of hybrid nanocarriers for the delivery of genes to various diseases. De Simon and his coworkers prepared the nanosized particles using the particle replication approach on the silicon wafers. The technique was referred to as Particle Replication in Nonwetting Templates (PRINT) [43]. The process involve the dissolution of the polymer (e.g., PLGA, PLA) in an organic solvents such as dimethyl formamide, methyl acetate and/or dimethyl sulfoxide along with the material to be encapsulated. The PRINT molding device was employed to fabricate the nanoparticles which later were harvested with the help of polyethylene terephthalate sheet [43]. It produces the particles of different shapes and a wide size range depending upon the size of the molding cavities [44].

2.3. Single-step preparation methods

The low encapsulation efficiency due to the leakage of the drugs from the inner core during second step, batch variability and large time consumption are the common problems associated with the conventional two step methods [45]. These constraints can be overcome by designing the simple method that utilized the single step approach and also provide better control on the content uniformity, reproducibility and other characteristics of the system. The method involves the mixing of two different solutions containing the polymer and lipid that self-assembled to form the particles with the core shell hybrid structure [46]. The polymer is dissolved in an appropriate organic solvent while the lipid solution is prepared in the water that may utilize the small fraction of organic solvent as solubilizing agent. The solution containing polymer is added to the lipid phase where the polymer precipitate to formed the nanoparticles and the lipid is self-assembled at the surface to form the hybrid nanoparticles. Single-step preparation is usually achieved by nanoprecipitation, emulsification-solvent evaporation and solvent diffusion methods. These methods and their appropriate modifications are discussed here.

2.3.1. Emulsification solvent evaporation method

Emulsification solvent evaporation method is the most commonly employed single step approach for the fabrication of hybrid nanocarriers. The single emulsification solvent evaporation [47] and double emulsification solvent evaporation (DESE) techniques are employed depending upon the nature and solubility of encapsulating drug. In the ESE method, the oil phase is formed by dissolving the polymer and the drug in the water immiscible organic solvent.

The aqueous solution containing the lipid portion which act as a stabilizer itself during the self-assembling process [48, 49]. The organic phase is then added dropwise into the aqueous phase under the sonication or stirring at the constant speed that results in the formation oil in water emulsion. During the emulsification process, the hydrophobic part of the lipid is adsorbed on the inner core material while the hydrophilic parts arrange themselves toward the aqueous medium forming the lipid coated hybrid nanoparticles [45, 50].

The single ESE method is employed for the encapsulation of hydrophobic drugs with low aqueous solubility [51]. Recently, the folate conjugated lipid polymer hybrid nanoparticles have been prepared by the emulsification solvent diffusion method for the targeted delivery of the doxorubicin using phosphatidylcholine (lecithin 99%) and 1,2-distearoyl-sn-glycero-3-phosphoethanolamine (DPSE)-PEG-COOH as lipid portion and PLGA as a polymeric portion [52]. The ESE method was also employed to formulate duel ligand hybrid nanocarriers for the targeted delivery of docetaxel. The hybrid nanoparticles possessed a uniform monolayer of the lipid over the polymeric core. The cell interaction studies revealed better endocytosis profile with sustained release of the drug by preventing the diffusion of the aqueous medium in the polymeric core. However, the particle were relative larger compared to that prepared by the nanoprecipitation method. This might be attributed to higher drug loading that maintained the therapeutic concentration for the longer period of time [53].

The double emulsification solvent evaporation (DESE) has been employed for the hydrophilic drugs and nucleic acid such as siRNA (small interfering ribonucleic acid) which are not dissolved in different organic solvents along with the other suitable polymers or the core/shell materials [54]. The aqueous solution of desired substance is prepared and is then emulsified in the organic/oil phase containing the lipid and polymer. The resultant primary emulsion is again added to another aqueous solution containing the lipid (lecithin, phosphatidylcholine or DSPE) or surface ligand (PEG, half antibodies, aptamer) and a water-in-oil-in-water (w/o/w) multiple emulsion is prepared. The evaporation of the organic phase results in the formation of hybrid nanoparticles [55]. The particles with hollow core covered with an appropriate shell provide the space for the internalization of hydrophilic and small molecules. The evaporation of the organic solvent provides the multilayered shell which has larger size as compared to the other methods [17].

Su et al. [56] prepared the reduction sensitive hybrid nanoparticles of doxorubicin using chitosan with the sodium dodecyl sulfate employing the double emulsification solvent evaporation method. The amphiphilic chitosan and lipid base micelles core provided a unique nanoconfiguration that is enveloped by the triglycerides which enhanced the loading efficiency and provided the drug release profile up to eight folds [56].

2.3.2. Nanoprecipitation

This method is also known as salting out method. It is a well known method for fabrication of hybrid nanoparticles of size less than 100 nm. This method employs two miscible solvents with different solubilizing capacity for the polymer. First, the polymer core is formed by solubilizing in solvent of greater solubility designated as good solvent which is then added to less soluble solvent designated as poor solvent. The two solutions are mixed by dropwise addition, stirring or sonication. Good solvent being miscible with poor solvent diffuses into later, leaving behind the core nanoparticles due to the precipitation of the polymer [19].

The core forming polymer and lipophilic drug are solubilized in a water-miscible organic solvent like acetone, acetonitrile or ethanol [57]. The lipids, inorganic salts or silica are dispersed in water with moderate heating (~60–75°C) and/or addition of hydroalcoholic mixtures for proper dispersion of the lipids.

The hydrophilic drugs are added to the aqueous phase containing dispersed lipids [58]. The polymer containing organic phase is then added dropwise to lipid dispersion with continuous stirring to precipitate the polymer into nanoparticles. The monodispersed hybrid nanoparticles are collected after suitable application of vortexing, homogenization or ultrasonication [55, 59]. Concurrent to the precipitation process, the self-assembly of lipid molecules around the polymer molecules occurs due to the hydrophobic interactions. The polymer core captures the hydrophobic tails of lipid while the heads are facing toward the aqueous phase [17, 60]. Continuous stirring of dispersion for several hours is helpful in uniform lipid coating of hybrid nanoparticles and to ensure the complete removal of organic solvent [55]. Rotary evaporator may also be helpful for the removal of organic solvents [58].

The literature suggests 10% ethanolic solution is employed for solubilization of lipids and PEG may enhance the stability of hybrid nanoparticles [61]. According to the study of Ling et al. [58], dextran sulfate and lecithin/PEG-PLGA hybrid nanoparticles can entrap higher amounts of hydrophilic moiety, the vincristine.

Wang et al. [62] developed PLGA/TPGS-lecithin hybrid nanoparticles using a modified nanoprecipitation method. The PLGA was dissolved in acetone while lipids were dispersed in either aqueous or 4% ethanolic aqueous solution. An inverse-phase nanoprecipitation method (i.e. aqueous phase was added dropwise into organic phase consisting of acetone, the PLGA and the paclitaxel). Initially, the formation of hybrid nanoparticles was slow due to the higher proportion of organic phase in the mixture. Continuous stirring and addition of water boosted the diffusion which leads to solidification of the hybrid nanoparticles. A stable hybrid nanoparticle formulation with low value of PDI (~0.1) was observed at 5:1 aqueous to organic phase ratio [62].

2.3.3. Sonication

Sonication is a fast technique for the fabrication of hybrid nanoparticles which utilizes ultrasonic waves rather than vortexing, solvent evaporation or heating. In this method, the two solutions designated as organic and aqueous phases lead to formation of inner core (polymer) and outer shell or coating materials (lipids), respectively. The sonication has been employed by Fang et al. [63] for the fabrication of hybrid nanoparticles of lecithin-PEG and PLGA by using this approach. The PLGA was dissolved in acetonitrile while the lecithin and the PEG were added in 4% ethanol solution. The former solution was carefully pipetted into the hydro alcoholic solution (aqueous to organic ratio was kept as 10:1). The hybrid nanoparticles were produced as this 'cocktail' mixture was placed in sonicator bath for five minutes at a frequency of 42 kHz and a power of 100 W. The main advantage of this technique is the formation of stable hybrid nanoparticles with short processing time and production rate is 20 times than other processes [63].

http://dx.doi.org/10.5772/66466

The sonication technique has been employed for PLGA and docetaxel hybrid nanoparticles by Liu et al. [64]. In another study, Mandal et al. [65] developed erlotinib loaded hybrid nanoparticles of PCL in which erlotinib and PCL were dissolved in acetone and added to the aqueous phase containing lipids. Hybrid nanoparticles were produced after sonication for 10 minutes at a frequency of 67 kHz and a power of 200 W [65].

A unique method using the combination of modified nanoprecipitation and sonication methods is presented for the fabrication of hybrid nanoparticles. In this method, the lipids melt was mixed with ethanolic solution of Elacridar, a chemosensitizer, and placed in vacuum oven until complete removal of solvents. The doxorubicin being hydrophilic drug was added in water with surfactant (Pluronic-F68) and heated (72–74°C). The drug and surfactant dispersion was mixed with Elacridar-lipid mixture. The whole mixture was stirred for 10 min and then ultrasonicated for two cycles of three minutes. It produced submicron sized lipid emulsion which was dispersed in 4–9 times higher volume of cold water (maintained 4°C) which leads to the formation of hybrid nanoparticles [66, 67].

2.3.4. Green technology for the preparation of hybrid nanocarriers

The use of green technology has revolutionized the synthesis of hybrid nanocarriers due to the ecofriendly procedures that mitigate the threats of toxic impurities and use of the organic solvents. These ecofriendly approaches also provided low operating cost, better stability, compatibility and minimum health hazards [68]. The literature has suggested the successful implementation of solvent free approaches to formulate nanosized systems for the targeted delivery of different therapeutic and diagnostic moieties.

The heat chill method has been employed to prepare micelles using the amphiphilic diblock and triblock copolymers of polycaprolactone (PCL) for the encapsulation of insulin without using any organic solvent and has provide better stability of the entrapped proteins which are liable to denaturation in the presence of different organic solvents [69].

Kumar et al. prepared the green PLGA-oil hybrid nanoparticles of resveratrol employing the acrysol oil (a derivative of castor oil) as nontoxic solvent. The nanoparticles have a smooth outer morphology with improved drug release and stability profile [70].

2.3.5. Preparation of organic/inorganic hybrid nanoparticles

The concept of combining the characteristics of organic and inorganic components is quite old since the time of Egyptian inks. However, the modern organic-inorganic hybrid systems are not prepared by simple mixing these materials but may involve the weak electrostatic linkages (H-bonding or van der Waals forces) or strong chemical bonds, i.e., covalent bonds [71]. Multiple strategies are employed for the preparation of these hybrid particles. These include (i) polymerization of the different monomers, organosilanes and the metal oxides, (ii) self-assembly of different structural components at nanoblock level with different organic and metal components, (iii) the functionalization of preformed nanocarriers with different organic compounds and (iv) making the core with organic materials and coating with the silica and different metallic components [72, 73].

Structural components	Physicochemical properties			Application	References
	Size (nm)	Zeta potential (mV)	Entrapment efficiency (%)		
PLA DPPC PEG-PE	278 ± 16	(+) 20 to 50	N/A	Steric stabilization of hybrid nanoparticles was enhanced at least up to 150 mM NaCl (for more than 1 year at 4°C).	[27]
Paclitaxel PLGA PEGylated octadecyl-quaternized lysine modified chitosan	194 ± 7	22 ± 4	87 ± 2	Folic acid modified polymer core lipid shell hybrid carrier for targeted anti-cancer therapy. Higher internalization up to 14.8 folds was observed in flow cytometry. It also showed higher cytotoxicity than commercial preparation (Taxol®). After 2 hours administration, it showed 3.70 fold higher bio distribution than Paclitaxel injection.	[39]
Levofloxacin Ciprofloxacin Ofloxacin PLGA Phosphatidylcholine (PC), Stearic Acid (SA)	420 260 360	-26 +26 -22	19 4 5	The amount of the polymer and lipid were optimized for highly efficient hybrid system. Hybrid nanoparticles showed higher size and drug encapsulation in comparison to polymeric carriers. Different antibiotics like levofloxacin, ciprofloxacin and ofloxacin were encapsulated. Ciprofloxacin showed less EE due to less lipophilicity. Oppositely charged drug and lipid prevented nanoparticle formation which was remedied by the addition of counter ionic surfactant.	[45]
Doxorubicin PLGA DEPE-PEG Lecithin	118.7 ± 0.75	15.19 ± 3.85	45.76 ± 6.58	Folate receptor mediated drug delivery of anti-cancer agent, doxorubicin, resulted in higher cell internalization and enhanced cell-killing effect toward MCF-7 cells with a significantly lower IC50.	[52]
PLGA DSPE-PEG Poly (β-aminoester) poly-1	280 ± 70	(+) 40 ± 7	N/A	mRNA loaded pH sensitive particles reached cytosol offering low cytotoxicity followed by translation at a frequency of ~30%. Intranasal administration of abovementioned system led to *in vivo* expression of protein as soon as 6 hours after administration.	[57]
Vincristine PLGA Poly ethylene glycol (PEG) Dextran sulfate	121.8–133	-8.5 to -14.6	64.7 to 93.6	Vincristine loaded hybrid nanocarriers resulted in 3.3-fold increase in apparent bioavailability, while its uptake was 12.4-fold higher than plain drug solution.	[58]

Structural components	Physicochemical properties			Application	References
	Size (nm)	Zeta potential (mV)	Entrapment efficiency (%)		
Docetaxel PLGA Lecithin PEG	70–80	-30 to -35	59 ± 4	Docetaxel loaded Hybrid nanoparticle exhibited 20 hourrs as T_{50}. These carriers also exhibited good stability in 10% bovine serum albumin and in 10% plasma solution.	[59]
Paclitaxel PLGA Soybean lecithin D-α-tocopheryl polyethylene glycol 1000 succinate (TPGS)	120–150	-15 to -20	>80	Developed carriers provided sustained release up to 8 days with a high tumor targeting potential through EPR effect. It also showed superior antitumor efficacy by inhibiting 58.8% volume of tumor at day 28.	[62]
PLGA DSPE-PEG	65	-47.7	N/A	A new quick single step preparation method is reported which needs 5 min to get accomplished. This method increased the production rate 20-fold without compromising determinant features of hybrid particles. Particles developed such exhibited good colloidal stability in PBS and serum over 5 days.	[63]
Docetaxel PLGA $DEPE-PEG_{2000}$	263.6	-20.74	66.88	Folic acid conjugation increased 38.2% for 0.5 hour incubation and 54% increase for 2 hours incubation during cell uptake study. Cell viability studies showed that formulation was 93.65% more effective than commercial preparation Taxotere®.	[64]
Erlotinib $DEPE-PEG_{2000}$ Dipalmitoylphosphatidylcholine (DPPC) N-[1-(2,3-Dioleoyloxy) propyl]-N,N,N-trimethylammonium methyl-sulfate (DOTAP)	161–271	-47	77.18	Erlotinib loaded Core Shell Lipid Polymer Hybrid Nanoparticles demonstrated 170 nm size with 66% Entrapment efficiency and greater uptake and efficiency in A549 cells.	[65]
Doxorubicin Elacridar Pluronic F-68	187–272	-19.7 to -22.9	71.2–89.3	Formulation shows up to 89% encapsulation efficiencies of Dox and GG918 in PLN with more uptake and cytotoxicity of Dox to MDR cells	[67]

Structural components	Physicochemical properties			Application	References
	Size (nm)	Zeta potential (mV)	Entrapment efficiency (%)		
Resveratrol PLGA	375 ± 13	-22 ± 1.6	76 ± 4.2	G-PONHs have higher biocompatibility and stability, but moderate cytotoxicity compared to standard NPs. It also involves the application green synthesis approach for the hybrid nanocarriers	[70]
Paclitaxel Poly-lactic-co-glycolic acid (PLGA) Soybean lecithin 1,2-Distearoyl-sn-glycero-3-phosphoethanolamine (DSPE-PEG)	186.9 ± 8.52	-29.5 ± 2.0	81.34 ± 3.41	More drug reaches target site crossing Blood brain barrier and survival time for mice was PtxR-FPLNs (42 days), Ptx-FPLNs (38 days) compared to PtxR (18 days) and Paclitaxal (14 days)	[76]
Melatonin Poly lactic acid (PLA) Didodecyldimethylammonium bromide (DDAB) Cetyltrimethylammonium bromide (CTAB)	180–218	+15.4 to -36.1	90.35	Coating with cationic lipids provides sustained and prolonged drug release, a pronounced benefit in ophthalmic application	[77]
Docetaxel PLGA DEPE-PEG_{2000} Soybean lecithin	60–70	-40 to -60	~62	The system provides 62% entrapment efficiency and almost 50% drug release in 20 hours. The incorporation of PEG provides stability over 120 hours. TC 50 value ranged between 4.58 and 5.55 mg.	[78]
PLGA DSPE-PEG	50–150	N/A	N/A	Different lipid ratios were evaluated for the entrapment, particle size, stability of the system. The current system provides that pH sensitive release and targeting which aggregate the drug in the acidic tumor microenvironment.	[79]
Poly caprolacton (PCL) Glyceryl tripalmitate	58–2009	-5.82 to -46.31	5.81–60.32	The system indicates biphasic release of the drug in which the burst release id presented in the initial hour. The cellular uptake was 83.3% in L929 cells. It also provides better colloidal stability over 120 hours.	[81]
Human IgG Poloxamer-188	135–799	+16.7 to +17.9	30.3–60	The system was loaded with the SiRNA. Which show the loading capacity of up to 2.04%, entrapment efficiency 60% in the optimized formulation. It provides the targetibility with the antibody and the sustain release was demonstrated by 20% release over the study time.	[82]

http://dx.doi.org/10.5772/66466

Structural components	Physicochemical properties			Application	References
	Size (nm)	Zeta potential (mV)	Entrapment efficiency (%)		
PCL Grape leaf extract Curcumin	~291	-24.3		The resulting drug delivery system improves the antimicrobial efficacy against two bacterial strains in addition to antifungal activity and can be an alternative approach to antibacterial agents.	[83]
Doxorubicin Epoxidized soybean oil Pluronic F68	200–350	-23.1	70 to 80	The system promotes cytotoxicity of DOX against MDR to about eightfolds. Uptake and retention of drug by MDR was also significantly increased.	[84]
Carboxymethyl chitosan Calcium phosphate PEG	102 ± 1.7	-8.25 ± 0.76	78	It gives excellent delivery of siRNA to cancer proximity through EPR effect. Particularly hTERT containing nanoparticles promotes silencing of hTERT expression and induction of cell apoptosis pathways.	[85]
Doxorubicin Sorafenib	126.3 ± 16.4	-21.4 ± 4.6	90.5 ± 3.4 and 70.8 ± 2.8	DOX-SOR combination in iRGD conjugated HNPs produces more apoptotic rates up to 44.7% than 33.4% with plain drug combinations or 37% with HNPs without iRGD.	[86]
Doxorubicin Mitomycin C	~150	~ -25	>90	Co delivery of anticancer agents using HNPs is more effective than simple combination therapy with advantages of high local delivery. It provides the 2–4 fold increase in the cellular uptake of the drug in the cancer cells.	[87]
Lipid modified PEG	24 ± 5	-38 ± 1	N/A	The system describes engineering of functionalized lipid conjugated polymeric nanoparticles with more specific targeting approach and imaging and bio sensing based on fluorescence.	[88]
Doxorubicin Combretastatin A4 PLGA PC DSPE-PEG Cholesterol	180–200	N/A	N/A	The system contains two different therapeutic agents which provide the site targeted release of the anti-angiogenesis agent and the anti-cancer drugs.	[89]
Curcumin PLGA DPPC DSPE-PEG	171.6 ± 8.2	N/A	N/A	By treating the metastatic breast cancer cells with the lipid-polymer hybrid nanoparticles of Curcumin decreased the adhesion onto tumor necrosis factor by 70% in capillary flow.	[90]

Structural components	Physicochemical properties			Application	References
	Size (nm)	Zeta potential (mV)	Entrapment efficiency (%)		
Docetaxel PLA Chitosan	208–255.7	-21.3 to + 52.4	75.9	PLA/chitosan nanoparticles provide rapid initial release of 40% drug in 5 hours and 70% cumulative release in 24 hours.	[91]
Docetaxel Curcumin PLGA	169.6 ± 4.6	-35.7 ± 1.9	89.8 ± 3.1 and 81.9 ±5.6	The drugs loaded hybrid nanoparticles showed enhanced cytotoxicity and tumor growth inhibition.	[92]
Docetaxel DSPE-PEG PLGA	110 ± 13.5	-25.67 ± 1.45	77.65 ± 0.57	The system increases the cellular update of docetaxel 2.5 folds and anti-proliferative activity 2.69–4.23 folds.	[93]
Doxorubicin Chitosan Hyaluronic acid	264 ± 2.2	-12.3 ± 2.0	97.8 ± 1.3	It is used to deliver anticancer drugs which results in enhanced circulation half-life and reduce the elimination of drug	[94]

Table 1. Hybrid nanoparticles with different structural components and their applications.

In conventional sol-gel approach, the hydrolysis process is used to obtain the hybrid system. The reaction involves the organically modified metal oxides which crosslinks with the polymers of multiple functionalities. These components may or may not be present in the organic solvents and possibly trapped within the inorganic material. However, use of self-assembling procedures in last few decades provided new methods for the fabrication. During the process, the inorganic materials (triblocks) were arranged by the use of organic surfactants. The preparation of the mesoporous hybrid with multiple functionalities provide highly porous surface which further modified based on the applications [74].

Shen and Shi [75] reported a method for preparation of the organic/inorganic hybrid based dendrimers. The metal or inorganic nanoparticles were entrapped in the dendrimers template to provide a modified surface morphology which can be tuned by different functional components to provide the biocompatibility and better colloidal stability [75] (**Table 1**).

3. Factors affecting hybrid nanocarriers

Hybrid nanoparticles are trimmed to an acceptable level of particle size, drug carrying capacity and site specificity through incorporation and adjustment of ratios of different chemical components. The variations of structural components of HNPs have an obvious influence on HNPs' characteristics [17, 96]. The principal factors of HNPs' formulation are (i) lipid/polymer ratio, (ii) PEGylation and (iii) polymer nature.

3.1. Lipid/polymer ratio

The lipid covering the polymeric core provides substantial benefits to HNPs and their distinction over nonhybrid nanoparticles. The ratio of two building blocks (lipid-polymer) of hybrid particles have significant role in stabilizing the formulation, monodispersibility and encapsulation efficiency [45, 97].

At a lower L/P ratio, the nanoparticle surfaces are not entirely covered with lipids, which can form bridges with lipid part of other particles causing aggregation and formation of larger particles. At a relative higher lipid concentration, it tends to decrease the production yield as whole amount is not incorporated in particles and free lipids will arrange themselves to form liposomes can affect the homogeneity of formulation. Therefore, the concentration of lipids should be optimized that cover to polymeric core on the basis of particle size and production yield [59, 98]. Chew et al. prepared HNPs with PC and PLGA carrying antibiotics with W_{PC}/W_{PLGA} value <15- up to 90%. At lipid amount below 15% larger particles were formed (800–1000 nm) and a sharp decrease in particle size was observed at an optimum concentration i.e. 30% lipids, an optimum particle size (260–400 nm) and 80% production yield was achieved. The lipid ratio above the optimum concentration i.e. 30% did not reduce particle size but it decreased the yield as the entire lipid was not utilized [45].

An optimum lipid to polymer ratio also provides the colloidal stability of HNPs by providing an optimum surface charge density which is responsible for electrostatic repulsive forces that prevent particle coalescence and stabilizes the formulation. In case where the lipid part is insufficient and the resulting electrostatic repulsive forces are weak, some agents like PEG can be incorporated in the formulations to provide steric repulsion and stabilization of the HNPs [52, 80–98].

The charge on lipid part which is responsible for electrostatic repulsion between particles is shielded when mixture of cationic and zwitterionic lipids is employed. Anionic heads of zwitterionic lipids face outwards which reduces of cationic lipids charge and promotes aggregation of particles. However, the higher cationic lipid concentration may overcome this charge screening and aggregation can be minimized [59, 99]. The zwitterionic lipid such as 1,2-dipalmitoyl-sn-glycero-3-phosphocholine (DPPC) produces less aggregation than a cationic lipid, 1,2-dipalmitoyl-3-trimethylammonium propane (DPTAP). Therefore, it zwitter ionic lipid provides more stability than ionic lipids [55, 59].

The two potential benefits that lipid augments to the HNPs are the encapsulation efficiency and retardant release of the incorporated drugs. The former is achieved by preventing drug leakage during self-assembling process, whereas the latter is due to reduced interaction of lipids with dissolution medium [17, 100]. The charge on the surface of lipids and drugs also affects the entrapment efficiency due to interaction of surface charge of HNPs and the charge of the drug. The loading of ciprofloxacin in the PLGA-PC hybrid system is not successful due to the interaction of cationic drug with the anionic lipids [19, 78].

A significant higher percent encapsulation of docetaxel (59 ± 4) was achieved in HNPs assembled from lecithin, DSPE-PEG and PLGA i.e. compared to PLGA-PEG nanoparticles with 19 ± 3 (mean ± SD). This effect is attributed to the fencing action of lipids which keeps hydrophobic drugs within the core and retards water penetration. The lipid-polymer hybrid formulations also provide a sustained release of drug when compared with nonhybrid formulation due to less water penetration and reduced escape of drug molecules from polymeric core. A consistent 50 % release of docetaxel from lecithin-PLGA hybrid system was observed compared to the PLGA-PEG NPs and PLGA NPs released same amount of drug in 10 hours and 7 hours, respectively. The pH of the dissolution media also affected the encapsulation of drugs, for example, the erlotinib EE % was 77.1%, 28.83% and 18.45% at pH values of 7.4, 5.4 and 3.4, respectively [55, 59, 78, 100].

3.2. PEGylation

The steric stabilization of HNPs systems to withstand salt solutions, buffer actions and uptake by macrophages is provided by the appropriate surface modification by employing PEG. The term is called as PEGylation. PEGs can escalate circulation times of HNPs by preventing particle aggregation, opsonization and adsorption of plasma proteins [27, 78].

Incorporation of PEG-lipid affects the colloidal stability of HNPs by two ways (i) chain length of PEG-lipid and (ii) molar Ratio of PEG-lipid. HNPs coated with PEG-lipid longer chains exhibited more stability than the shorter chain PEG-lipid coated particles. Similarly, at the fixed chain length more PEG-lipid incorporated onto polymer core and thickness of lipid shell increased which lowered the zeta potential and hence stability is enhanced [78, 80].

Yang et al. studied the effect of lipid/polymer ratio and PEGylation on HNPs prepared from PLA/mPEG-PLA polymer and BHEM-Chol cationic lipid. HNPS prepared from mPEG-PLA were smaller and more stable in PBS at the given lipid/polymer ratio than PLA alone [61].

Fang et al. formulated HNPs using 0.10–0.35 lipid-PEG/PLGA ratios without incorporating lecithin. Initially particle reduced with increase in lipid amount and optimized at 0.30 lipid-PEG/PLGA ratio after which further increase in lipids did not affect particle size and PDI. At an optimized (0.30 lipid-PEG/PLGA) ratio, lipid-PEG was replaced with mole equivalents of lecithin. The stable particles of 60 nm were obtained at 50% lipid-PEG replacement. Upon 70% lipid-PEG replacement, the size was increased to 100 nm and at 80% lipid-PEG replacement with lecithin, the unstable particles were obtained. This instability of particles is due to the replacement of higher lipid-PEG content, a major stability component of HNPs [63].

3.3. Nature of polymer

The characteristics such as density and surface charge play an important role in the fabrication of HNPs [35]. The density of polymer also has substantial effect on stability and particle size [59, 78]. HNPs fabricated from high density polymer are less stable toward increasing ionic strength of medium due to the higher sedimentation rate when electrostatic charges are shielded. PLA is 1.18 times denser than poly(styrene); hence, HNPs prepared with PLA core have less colloidal stability toward increasing ionic strength of medium [35]. Zhang et al. evaluated that change in viscosity of PLGA polymer from 0.19 to 0.82 resulted a decrease in particle diameter from 92.7 nm to 66.7 nm [59].

Adsorption of lipid over polymeric particle surface to form lipid shell depends upon curvature and surface charge of particle. Cationic lipids exhibit more adsorption than zwitter ions toward the anionic polymeric core due to the electrostatic attractions polymeric core from anionic polymer PLA has greater affinity for DPTAP cationic lipid than the zwitterionic DPPC. Lipid rearrangement around polymeric core can be quick and complete if the affinity between polymer and lipid is high. Larger size distribution and free lipid structures are observed when lipids cannot rearrange around polymeric core due to weaker affinity. Modification in pH of medium can improve the affinity of polymer for lipid by surface charge variation at different pH levels [35, 101, 102].

4. Applications of hybrid nanocarriers

Hybrid systems combine properties of two or more materials, thus, appear superior to individual material system. Usually, one component of hybrid system is active, whereas other is used to improve biocompatibility, circulation life and targeting. Many new hybrid systems use second material to improve efficiency of first materials. By suitable selection of materials, hybrid systems find wider applications in medical field. Hydrophilic polymers have been widely used to impart stealth property to nanoparticles. However, stealth coating does not improve or impart new functional aspect of nanoparticles. Thus, many researchers do not regard PEG coated as hybrid systems. Similarly, nanoparticles conjugated with targeting ligands cannot be regarded as hybrid system.

4.1. Lipid polymer hybrid nanoparticles (LPHN)

LPHN consists of a drug containing polymeric core which is coated by a lipid shell. In these systems, inner polymer core contains drug and lipid shell is used to enhance penetration through biological membranes and to control drug release. Polymeric core can be made from hydrophilic or hydrophobic polymer. Term lipid-polymer hybrid is also used for systems that contain polymer core with lipid coating. Lipid is preferred carrier material for hydrophobic drugs due to higher encapsulation efficiency and extended release pattern. A polymeric coating is applied over lipid core to impart certain characteristics required for novel biomedical applications.

In addition of polymeric and lipid layers, surface of LPHN may be modified with different materials. In one study, a hydrophobic drug was loaded in a hydrophobic biodegradable polymer to enhance encapsulation efficiency of a hydrophobic drug. Then, a lipid layer is applied to stabilize core and shell, and to prolong drug release. Finally, hydrophilic polymeric layer, consisting of DSPE-PEG (1,2-distearoyl-sn-glycero-3-phosphoethanolamine-N-carboxy (polyethylene glycol)2000) was applied to improve pharmacokinetics of LPHN. The three-layer LPHN showed high encapsulation and sustained release of hydrophilic drug [59]. A hydrophilic polymer monolayer may be applied to LPHN to escape phagocytosis and early removal from body. Generally, polyethylene glycol (PEG) is used to provide this stealth property and enhance circulation time of nanoparticles. PEG will attract water to make an aqueous layer which protect LPHN from attachment of opsonin proteins and let it escape the uptake by reticuloendothelial (RES) system. Hydrophilic polymer layer can also enhance colloidal stability of LPHN due to steric hindrance effect [5]. As stealth layer can also hinder interaction with target cells, PEG can be conjugated with other monomers or polymers to form block copolymers that are specific to certain stimuli. This approach enables long circulating LPHN that can shed stealth layer when come in contact with target cells. The stimuli could be intracellular and extracellular protease enzymes, low pH or reducing agents [103].

Selection of polymeric matrix plays a major role in drug delivery properties of LPHN. LPHN are commonly used for poor water soluble or hydrophobic drugs. A hydrophobic polymer core can encapsulate higher amount of hydrophobic drug and vice versa. Two or more drugs could also be loaded into the core of LPHN. On the other hand, LPHN with hydrophilic and hydrophobic drug could be made to contain one drug in core and the other in shell. Wong et al. [67] prepared LPHN containing lipid core to encapsulate hydrophobic drug Elacridar (GG918) and hydrophilic shell of hydrolyzed polymer of epoxidized soybean oil (HPESO) to encapsulated doxorubicin. They found that both drugs were released in sustained manner for more than 72 hours (**Figure 2**). Simultaneous delivery of chemosensitizer GG918 was able to revert multidrug resistance to anticancer drug doxorubicin. These simultaneously loaded LPHN showed better efficacy than free drug solution or LPHN of any of the two drugs.

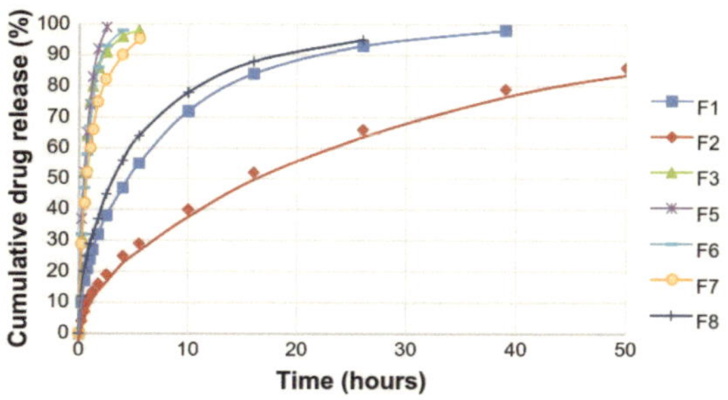

Figure 2. Drug release from gold nanoparticles containing solid lipid nanoparticles. F1 (5mg diacerein) and F2 (10 mg diacerein) show sustained release of drug for 39 and 48 hours. However, F3 had same composition as F2 but drug release was conducted at 40°C. F5 and F6 contained increasing amount of hydrophilic gold nanoparticles with 5 mg diacerein. F7 contained gold nanoparticles same as F6 but 10 mg diacerein. Finally, F8 contained lipophilic gold nanoparticles with 10 mg diacerein. Drug release was faster at higher temperature (F3) as compared to 37°C. Furthermore, hydrophilic gold nanoparticles containing formulations F5, F6 and F7 released drug in less than 5 hours, whereas hydrophobic gold nanoparticles showed prolonged release up to 25 hours.

As a wide variety of polymers and lipids are available, LPHN can be prepared to theoretically load any therapeutic moiety. Nucleic acid based therapeutics i.e. plasmid DNA, antisense oligonucleotide, small interfering RNA and small hairpin RNA, have shown promise to cure many diseases. LPHN have emerged as nonviral carriers for nucleic acid products with low toxicity, immunogenicity and cost of production. Cationic polymers and lipids have been widely investigated for this purpose. Cationic groups can bind negatively charged nucleic acid molecules and deliver to target cells. Zhong et al. [104] prepared LPHN with biodegradable PLGA and two cationic lipids i.e. 1, 2-dioleoyl-3-trimethyammonium-propane (DOTAP) or 3β-[N-(N′,N′-dimethylaminoethane)-carbamyl]cholesterol (DC-Chol). LPHN were prepared by two either with cationic lipid core so that DNA is loaded inside core or with cationic lipid shell so that DNA is loaded on surface. The *in vitro* evaluation was done in human embryonic kidney cells. They found that LPHN with DNA on surface showed higher transfection efficiency than those with DNA inside core. Next, they prepared LPHN with polymer both inside core and on the surface which showed efficiency similar to that of LPHN with DNA on surface. This study concluded that LPHN can show transfection efficiency about 600 times higher than unbound DNA. However, cationic lipids and polymers may have some problems on their own. They may interact with biological components, be nonbiodegradable or toxic after systemic administration. These factors are controlled by hydrophobic chain length, nature of cation group and linkage. To solve these problems, Shi et al. [54] prepared novel LPHN with four distinct layers. First is a hollow core i.e. aqueous droplet containing nucleic acid which is coated by an inner lipid layer of cationic lipid ethylphosphocholine.

The cationic lipid orients itself in such a way that cationic group faces inward and its hydrophobic chain faces outward. Third layer is formed by ester terminated PLGA. It is a hydrophobic polymer that intermingles with protruding chains of cationic lipid. Finally, self-assembled lecithin and DSPE-PEG form outer coating to facilitate transfection and to impart stealth property to LPHN. This LPHN system release loaded siRNA in sustained manner up to 6 days and enhanced gene expression in mice.

A recent trend in drug delivery research has focused on the development of human-like vesicular drug delivery system. This concept emerged when exosome were found to be responsible for cell to cell communication in tumors and regulate tumor microenvironment. It was believed that exosomes isolated from patients may be filled with antitumor drugs and injected back to the patients for personalized treatment. As isolation of exosomes from patients is complicated and very costly, this dream was realized by synthesizing surface antigens of exosomes by genetic engineering and grafting on the surface of drug containing liposomes or other vesicular systems [5]. In addition to this, many bacterial and viral antigens have been used. These antigens are used for the delivery of vaccine and act as immune adjuvant i.e. enhance immune response to vaccine. Moreover, polymeric core produce better adjuvant effects than lipid core. Bershteyn et al. [105] prepared PLGA core and phospholipid bilayer coated LPHN that were stabilized by PEG for simultaneous loading of antigen and adjuvant. The protein adjuvant was covalently bonded on surface and lipophilic adjuvants, such as monophosphoryl lipid A and α-galactosylceramide, which were loaded in lipid bilayer. Immune response was shown at dose as low as 2.5 ng which was detectable after 100 days. It was also found that α-galactosylceramide shows rapid rise in antibody titer whereas monophosphoryl lipid A produced response in sustained manner. Interestingly, coloading of both adjuvants with antigen further increased antigen titer by 12 fold. These results show that LPHN can reduce dose of antigen to reduce cost and side effects.

Term LPHN may also be extended to nanoparticle systems consisting of two or more polymer at least one of which is lipophilic. A hydrophilic shell may be applied to drug containing hydrophobic (or lipophilic) polymeric core to impart mucoadhesion or to make them stealth. For example, PEG or chitosan coating has been widely used to improve circulation life of sustained release solid lipid nanoparticles [106]. On the other hand, a hydrophobic polymer shell may be formed over hydrophilic polymer core to enhance LPHN absorption through biological membranes. This approach is especially useful for oral administration of therapeutic macromolecules [107]. Recently, Liu et al. has synthesized supramolecular vectors for gene delivery. First, adamantyl-terminated polyethyleneimine was admixed with β-cyclodextrin to encapsulate nucleic acid, i.e., DNA or siRNA which was further coated with adamantyl-PEG. The supramolecular vector was stabilized by host-guest interaction. This LPHN system showed low toxicity and high transfection efficiency during in vitro experiments. Graphene is another two-dimensional framework of carbon atoms that is investigated for hybrid applications. When treated with suitable reagents, it can be oxidized, hydroxylated, carboxylated or halogenated. These functional groups can be conjugated with different materials desired for biomedical applications [108].

4.2. Inorganic/organic hybrid nanoparticles (IOHN)

IOHN are synthesized from organic and inorganic materials. Most commonly, core is made of inorganic materials and the shell of an organic material is applied to improve its pharmacokinetic parameters. On the other hand, inorganic shell may be applied to the core of organic materials to impart different properties. IOHN are interesting because they offer properties of both materials. Like organic polymer, they can be functionalized with different groups. Like metallic nanoparticles, inorganic shell provides physical and chemical stability to polymeric core. Generally, the inorganic portion is developed by reduction of metal ions to zerovalent state. Inorganic core is synthesized by mixing metal ions solution with a reducing agent with or without heating. However, inorganic shell may be synthesized either by reduction of metal ions on polymeric core or by deposition of preformed metal colloids on organic core.

Methods for synthesis of organic core and shell have already been discussed in detail in a chapter. We have prepared IOHN consisting of gold core with fatty acid shell. First, gold nanoparticles were synthesized with lecithin bilayer (hydrophilic surface) and lecithin monolayer by acid treatment (hydrophobic surface). The gold nanoparticles were added to molten fatty acids and emulsified with aqueous surfactant solution. Upon cooling, we found that gold nanoparticles with hydrophobic surface are more stable as compared to gold nanoparticles with hydrophilic surface [109]. The presence of gold nanoparticles in core enhanced drug release rate from lipid nanoparticles. This can be attributed to the presence of gold nanoparticles that push drug toward periphery and reduce diffusion path length (**Figure 1**). In another study, we prepared an organic core of lecithin and inorganic shell of gold nanoparticles. First, lecithin nanoparticles were prepared and loaded with drug. Next, preformed gold nanoparticles were adsorbed on its surface. We found that drug release was controlled by both gold nanoparticles. Gold nanoparticles retard release of drug due to physical barrier. Lecithin controlled release of anti-inflammatory drug from core in pH-dependent manner [110]. Gold is also known to possess anti-inflammatory effect. In this study, gold shell was found to synergize anti-inflammatory effect of encapsulated drug diacerein by many folds (**Figure 3**).

Various organic materials have been used to prepare IOHN to improve their performance. The materials that are used to synthesize or stabilize nanoparticles may impart specific function. The most pronounced function is enhanced penetration inside target cells which in turn controls toxicity of IOHN. Freese et al. [47] studied toxicity of gold nanoparticles with different organic coatings with neutral, positive and negative charge. The results showed that IOHN with positive charge coating shows more internalization in cells, and thus, higher toxicity. The cell membrane has a negative charge, whereas the IOHN are positively charged particles. This charge difference triggers the rapid binding to the cell surface and internalization of these IOHNs. As gold can cause toxicity at higher dose, higher internalization in cell will lead to high toxicity [111].

Metallic nanoparticles smaller than 100 nm are usually responsive to different stimuli, a technique that has been widely employed in diagnosis and therapy. IOHN with metallic core can be used for thermotherapy of cancer whereby IOHN produces heat when exposed to external magnetic field. Similarly, metallic moieties, i.e., nanoparticles or tagged polymers, can be bound to core of organic materials. These nanoparticles will be targeted to cancerous tissues and magnetic moieties will produce hyperthermia under external stimuli. When core of organic material is loaded with drug, inorganic part can release the drug by hyperthermia-mediated degradation of core after reaching the target site [5]. In addition to magnetic field, inorganic nanoparticles are also responsive to infrared and ultrasound waves. This makes IOHN interesting candidates for biomedical imaging of targeted tis-

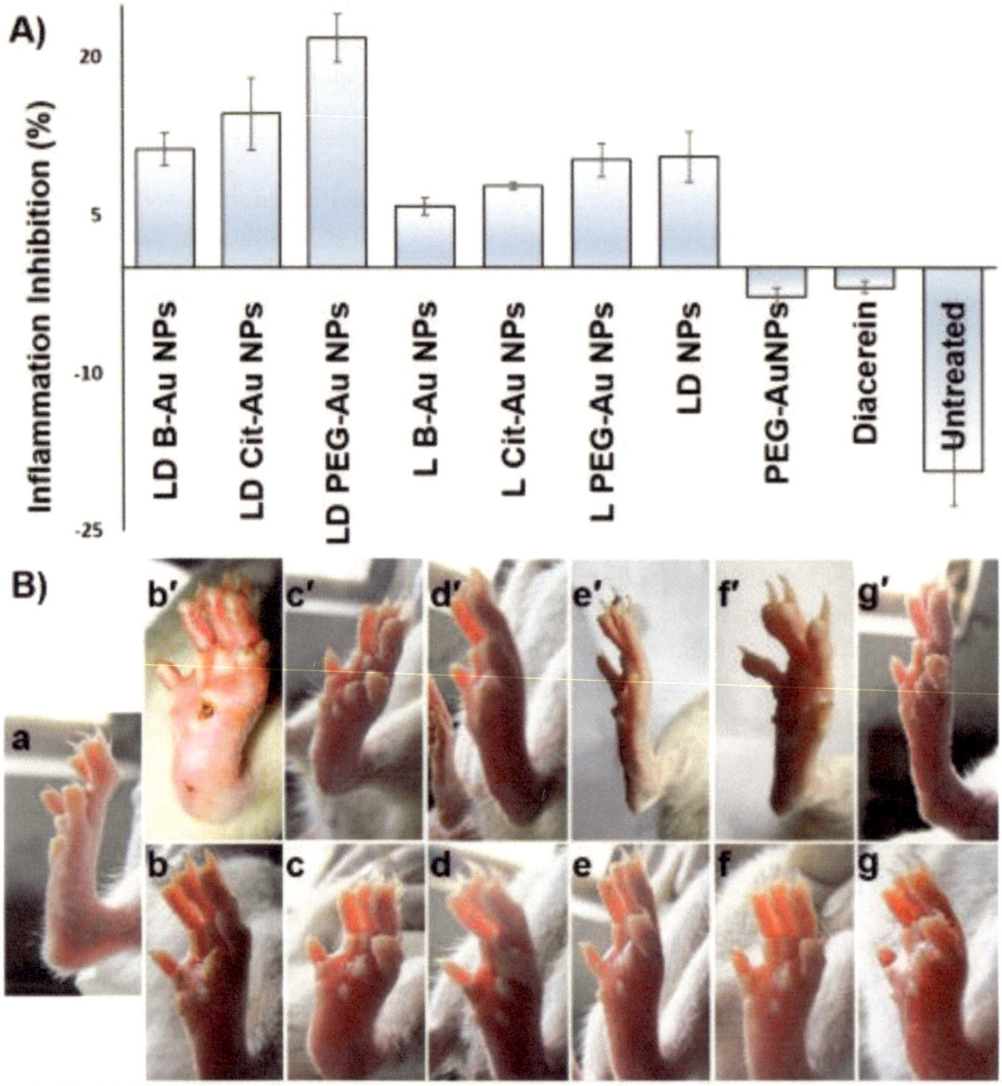

Figure 3. Efficacy of anti-inflammatory drug encapsulated in lecithin core-gold shell hybrid nanoparticles; (A) Anti-inflammatory effect of diacerein is synergized in the presence of gold as compared to pure drug, diacerein. PEG-AuNP = PEG coated gold nanoparticles, LD-NP = diacerein loaded lecithin nano[articles, L PEG-AuNP = Lecithin nanoparticles surface coated with PEG coated gold nanoparticles, L Cit-AuNP = Lecithin nanoparticles surface coated with citrate coated gold nanoparticles, L B-AuNP = Lecithin nanoparticles surface coated with sodium borohydrate coated gold nanoparticles, LD PEG-AuNP = L PEG-AuNP loaded with diacerein, LD Cit-AuNP = L Cit-AuNP loaded with diacerein, LD B-AuNP = L B-AuNP loaded with diacerein. (B) represents decrease in swelling as measured by Vernier caliper before (a, b, c, d, e, f, g) and 3 h after (b′,c′, d′, e′, f′, g′) from untreated (b), diacerein (c), PEG-Au NPs (d), LD PEG-Au NPs (e), LD Cit-Au NPs (f), and LD B-Au NPs (g) treatments groups, while a is normal rat paw.

sues. More recently, multimodal IOHN have ensured imaging and drug release from the same system after systemic administration. This target can be achieved in two ways. First, magnetic field of low frequency or intensity is applied for imaging of IOHN. Once in cancer tissue, intensity or frequency is increased to produce hyperthermia-based cell killing or drug release [112]. Secondly, inorganic materials responsive to more than one stimulus can be used. One stimulus aids in imaging, whereas second stimulus will lead to drug release or thermotherapy [113].

IOHN have also been prepared with hollow core enclosed inside a hybrid shell. Hollow core IOHN can be prepared by many ways. First strategy is to make layer of inorganic or organic material which is then stabilized by other component of IOHN system. Similarly, it can consist of a mixed shell of inorganic and organic materials enclosing hollow core. Metal-tagged polymers with amphiphilic nature self-assemble to form micelles in aqueous solution or after reaching the target microenvironment [114]. Whole virus or virus capsid has been investigated as drug delivery systems by many researchers due to its inherent high penetration in cells.

Portney et al. [115] hybridized virus capsid with quantum dots and single-wall carbon nanotubes to yield hybrid structures that can find various applications. These hybrid structures are very stable to chemical and mechanical stress. IOHN with metallic core and organic shells have been widely investigated for diagnostic application. Although, organic shell usually employed to improve the pharmacokinetics and targeting properties of the metallic nanoparticles but may be beneficial by enhancing the diagnostic efficiency of the system. The most prominent example is nucleic acid-based biosensors with metallic core. When metallic nanoparticles aggregate, they show blue shift due to increase in size. Metallic core is coated with single-stranded DNA (ssDNA) that can identify specific sequence on target DNA and bind it. In bioassay, when metallic nanoparticle conjugated ssDNA start bind target DNA, they come close to each other and test solution color changes from red to blue. This indicates the presence of target DNA as visualized by naked eye or through UV-visible spectrophotometer [116].

4.3. Metalloprotein hybrid nanoflowers (MPHNs)

Although MPHN can be categorized as inorganic-organic hybrid NP, they are discussed here separately due to difference in structure and many fold increased surface area. The flower-like structure of MPHN is due to the presence of proteins that stabilize metallic crystals in the structure. Proteins act as glue and hold metallic crystals in a pattern which mimics flower petals. Unlike inorganic-organic hybrids, synthesis of MPHN occurs in three stages. First stage is the growth stage in which metal ions bond with proteins through amide bond. This acts as nucleation site leading to growth of primary crystals. In the second stage, metalloprotein crystals aggregate to form larger structures bearing primary petals like structures. Finally, anisotropic growth on metalloprotein aggregates leads to formation of complete petals. Generally, their size lies in the range of 2–30 μm which is another reason to differentiate MPHN from OIHN. MPHN is mostly used for bioassay whereby desired enzyme is conjugated with metallic part. Encapsulation efficiency of enzymes in MPHN has been achieved up to 66%. Enzyme loading above or below this limit decreases encapsulation efficiency. Nevertheless, enzyme efficiency of MPHN varies between 85% and 1000%. Enzyme efficiency higher than free enzyme is due to many reasons. MPHN shows high surface area due to petal-like projections. The petals also have hole-like spaces between them that may be up to 100 nm in diameter. It is also observed that immobilized enzyme shows cooperative interaction to enhance enzyme efficiency. Similarly, metal ions, such as copper, calcium and manganese, may also help enzyme in catalysis. Copper (Cu^{2+}) is the most widely used metal with different enzymes. Cu^{2+} and laccase enzyme MPHN have been developed for detection of phenols. The prepared MPHN was adsorbed on filter, and a mixture of phenol and 4-aminoantipyrine was added to it. Laccase-assisted reaction of both compounds produced red antipyrine dyes in 5 minutes. The changes in color will be visible with the naked eye, and UV-visible spectrophotometer can be used for quantitative detection. The MPHN-coated filters are reusable and are much faster than chromatography and mass spectrometry based methods. Likewise, MPHN of Cu^{2+} and horseradish peroxidase was prepared for detection of phenol and hydrogen peroxide. This MPHN was able to detect very low amounts of phenol (1 μM) and hydrogen peroxide (0.5 μM) as change in color was observed with the naked eye. It has been found that hydrogen peroxide induces cell death at concentration higher than 50 μM and the limit of detection of free enzyme is around 20 μM. Thus, these MPHNs will be very efficient to detect slight changes in hydrogen peroxide efficiently even below its threshold level. Cu^{2+} and trypsin MPHN have been used to carry out proteolysis which is an important step in protein identification. The enzyme efficiency of proteolytic MPHN is similar or superior to free enzyme but are fast and reusable.

Another form of nanoflowers is synthesized using deoxyribonucleic acid (DNA) which, like proteins, possesses high number of nitrogen molecules and serves as a template for nanoflowers. In one study, a drug and a dye molecule was bonded to DNA that was used to synthesize nanoflowers. These nanoflowers showed multimodel property of drug delivery and imaging by using FRET technology. More recently, capsular MPHNs have been prepared with improved characteristics. This technique involved coating of MPHN with protamine and silica. Then, metallic core is removed from capsular MPHN system. Capsular nanoflowers show higher enzyme efficiency and improved stability in harsh environmental conditions.

4.4. Mesoporous silica hybrid nanoparticles

Silica has been widely used in drug delivery due to its nontoxic and biocompatible nature. Silica shell has been applied to metallic nanoparticles to reduce their toxicity in various biomedical applications. Mesoporous silica nanoparticles (MSNPs) are silica materials with mesopores of up to 50 nm. They are also termed as hollow mesoporous silica nanoparticles due to the fact that mesopores are hollow. The advantages of MSNP are enhanced surface area and that hollow mesopores can be loaded with therapeutic molecules. First, MSNPs were loaded with drugs. Later, MSNPs were used for the delivery of different dyes and macromolecules such as enzymes. MSNP hybrids have been prepared with both organic and inorganic materials. One problem with the use of MSNP is the leakage of drugs from pores. Sreejith et al. [117] used graphene oxide (GO) coating on MSNP to prevent leakage of drugs. After drug loading, GO coating is applied which acts as blanket to physically block the pores. GO coating also prevents encapsulated drug from environmental degradation. In addition to applications in drug delivery, MSNPs are also used for diagnosis and imaging.

Maji et al. [118] prepared MSNP-GNP (gold nanoparticle) hybrids for detection of hydrogen peroxide. They coated MSNP with graphene oxide, and GNPs were coated on this surface.

The hybrids were first used for electrochemical detection of hydrogen peroxide in the presence of other biological molecules. Later, MSNP-GNPs were successfully used for in vivo imaging in mice. MSNP surface can be modified with different functional groups that provide opportunities to form hybrid with different materials [118].

5. Conclusion and future prospects

Hybrid nanocarriers provide a novel platform that synergizes the effects of therapeutic and diagnostic agents through tunable properties such as particle size, structure, composition, preparatory method and easy surface and charge modifications. Here, we describe the different parameters related to development, optimization as well as characterization to obtain a robust platform for the drug delivery and other biomedical applications. We can still try to focus some unmet challenges of this novel drug delivery system. These challenges include development and optimization of the application of target ligands in appropriate ligand density that will improve the pharmacokinetics as well as pharmacodynamics profiles of all the drugs loaded in these hybrid nanoparticles either single or in combination with other therapeutic and diagnostic agents. Similarly, development of these hybrid nanocarriers at large scale has received less attention. So it is a key parameter to translate the system for large-scale applications by using the different methods mentioned in the section of method of preparation especially the one-step self-assembly method that is likely to improve the production in a facile and economic manner.

Author details

Asadullah Madni*, Nayab Tahir, Mubashar Rehman, Ahmed Raza, Muhammad Ahmad Mahmood, Muhammad Imran Khan and Prince Muhammad Kashif

*Address all correspondence to: asadpharmacist@hotmail.com

Faculty of Pharmacy and Alternative Medicine, The Islamia University of Bahawalpur, Bahawalpur, Pakistan

References

[1] Li M, Luo Z, Zhao Y. Hybrid nanoparticles as drug carriers for controlled chemotherapy of cancer. The Chemical Record. 2016. DOI: 10.1002/tcr.201600029.

[2] Gong J, Chen M, Zheng Y, Wang S, Wang Y. Polymeric micelles drug delivery system in oncology. Journal of Controlled Release. 2012;159(3):312–323. DOI: 10.1016/j.jconrel.2011.12.012.

[3] Mieszawska AJ, Kim Y, Gianella A, van Rooy I, Priem B, Labarre MP, et al. Synthesis of polymer–lipid nanoparticles for image-guided delivery of dual modality therapy. Bioconjugate Chemistry. 2013;24(9):1429–1434. DOI: 10.1021/bc400166j.

[4] Mehnert W, Mäder K. Solid lipid nanoparticles: production, characterization and applications. Advanced Drug Delivery Reviews. 2001;47(2):165–196. DOI: 10.1016/S0169-409X(01)00105-3.

[5] Madni A, Sarfraz M, Rehman M, Ahmad M, Akhtar N, Ahmad S, et al. Liposomal drug delivery: a versatile platform for challenging clinical applications. Journal of Pharmacy & Pharmaceutical Sciences. 2014;17(3):401–426. DOI: http://dx.doi.org/10.18433/J3CP55.

[6] Fan J, Fang G, Wang X, Zeng F, Xiang Y, Wu S. Targeted anticancer prodrug with mesoporous silica nanoparticles as vehicles. Nanotechnology. 2011;22(45):455102.

[7] Prabaharan M, Grailer JJ, Pilla S, Steeber DA, Gong S. Gold nanoparticles with a monolayer of doxorubicin-conjugated amphiphilic block copolymer for tumor-targeted drug delivery. Biomaterials. 2009;30(30):6065–6075. DOI: 10.1016/j.biomaterials.2009.07.048.

[8] Torchilin V. Multifunctional and stimuli-sensitive pharmaceutical nanocarriers. European Journal of Pharmaceutics and Biopharmaceutics. 2009;71(3):431–444. DOI: 10.1016/j.ejpb.2008.09.026.

[9] Krishnamurthy S, Vaiyapuri R, Zhang L, Chan JM. Lipid-coated polymeric nanoparticles for cancer drug delivery. Biomaterials Science. 2015;3(7):923–936. DOI: 10.1039/C4BM00427B

[10] He Y, Zhang L, Song C. Luteinizing hormone-releasing hormone receptor-mediated delivery of mitoxantrone using LHRH analogs modified with PEGylated liposomes. International Journal of Nanomedicine 2010;5:697–705. DOI: 10.2147/IJN.S12129.

[11] Zhang L, Zhu D, Dong X, Sun H, Song C, Wang C, et al. Folate-modified lipid–polymer hybrid nanoparticles for targeted paclitaxel delivery. International Journal of Nanomedicine 2015;10:2101–2114. DOI: 10.2147/IJN.S77667.

[12] Lee S-M, Ahn RW, Chen F, Fought AJ, O'halloran TV, Cryns VL, et al. Biological evaluation of pH-responsive polymer-caged nanobins for breast cancer therapy. ACS Nano. 2010;4(9):4971–4978. DOI: 10.1021/nn100560p.

[13] Montasser I, Shahgaldian P, Perret F, Coleman AW. Solid lipid nanoparticle-based calix [n] arenes and calix-resorcinarenes as building blocks: synthesis, formulation and characterization. International Journal of Molecular Sciences. 2013;14(11):21899–21942. DOI: 10.3390/ijms141121899.

[14] Liechty WB, Kryscio DR, Slaughter BV, Peppas NA. Polymers for drug delivery systems. Annual Review of Chemical and Biomolecular Engineering. 2010;1:149. DOI: 10.1146/annurev-chembioeng-073009-100847.

[15] Reis CP, Neufeld RJ, Ribeiro AJ, Veiga F. Nanoencapsulation I. Methods for preparation of drug-loaded polymeric nanoparticles. Nanomedicine: Nanotechnology, Biology and Medicine. 2006;2(1):8–21. DOI: 10.1016/j.nano.2005.12.003.

[16] Zheng M, Yue C, Ma Y, Gong P, Zhao P, Zheng C, et al. Single-step assembly of DOX/ICG loaded lipid–polymer nanoparticles for highly effective chemo-photothermal combination therapy. ACS Nano. 2013;7(3):2056–2067. DOI: 10.1021/nn400334y.

[17] Hadinoto K, Sundaresan A, Cheow WS. Lipid–polymer hybrid nanoparticles as a new generation therapeutic delivery platform: a review. European Journal of Pharmaceutics and Biopharmaceutics. 2013;85(3):427–443. DOI: 10.1016/j.ejpb.2013.07.002.

[18] Qi D, Cao Z, Ziener U. Recent advances in the preparation of hybrid nanoparticles in miniemulsions. Advances in Colloid and Interface Science. 2014;211:47–62. DOI: 10.1016/j.cis.2014.06.001.

[19] Zhang L, Zhang L. Lipid–polymer hybrid nanoparticles: synthesis, characterization and applications. Nano Life. 2010;1(1):163–173. DOI: 10.1142/S179398441000016X.

[20] Hu C-MJ, Zhang L, Aryal S, Cheung C, Fang RH, Zhang L. Erythrocyte membrane-camouflaged polymeric nanoparticles as a biomimetic delivery platform. Proceedings of the National Academy of Sciences. 2011;108(27):10980–10985. DOI: 10.1073/pnas.1106634108.

[21] Allen TM, Cullis PR. Liposomal drug delivery systems: from concept to clinical applications. Advanced Drug Delivery Reviews. 2013;65(1):36–48. DOI: 10.1016/j.addr.2012.09.037.

[22] Zhang L, Granick S. How to stabilize phospholipid liposomes (using nanoparticles). Nano Letters. 2006;6(4):694–698. DOI: 10.1021/nl052455y.

[23] Mieszawska AJ, Gianella A, Cormode DP, Zhao Y, Meijerink A, Langer R, et al. Engineering of lipid-coated PLGA nanoparticles with a tunable payload of diagnostically active nanocrystals for medical imaging. Chemical Communications. 2012;48(47):5835–5837. DOI: 10.1039/C2CC32149A.

[24] Jain S, Valvi PU, Swarnakar NK, Thanki K. Gelatin coated hybrid lipid nanoparticles for oral delivery of amphotericin B. Molecular Pharmaceutics. 2012;9(9):2542–2553. DOI: 10.1021/mp300320d.

[25] Kamaly N, Xiao Z, Valencia PM, Radovic-Moreno AF, Farokhzad OC. Targeted polymeric therapeutic nanoparticles: design, development and clinical translation. Chemical Society Reviews. 2012;41(7):2971–3010. DOI: 10.1039/C2CS15344K.

[26] Nicolas J, Mura S, Brambilla D, Mackiewicz N, Couvreur P. Design, functionalization strategies and biomedical applications of targeted biodegradable/biocompatible polymer-based nanocarriers for drug delivery. Chemical Society Reviews. 2013; 42(3):1147–1235. DOI: 10.1039/C2CS35265F.

[27] Thevenot J, Troutier A-L, David L, Delair T, Ladavière C. Steric stabilization of lipid/polymer particle assemblies by poly (ethylene glycol)-lipids. Biomacromolecules. 2007;8 (11):3651–3660. DOI: 10.1021/bm700753q.

[28] De Miguel I, Imbertie L, Rieumajou V, Major M, Kravtzoff R, Betbeder D. Proofs of the structure of lipid coated nanoparticles (SMBV™) used as drug carriers. Pharmaceutical Research. 2000;17(7):817–824. DOI: 10.1023/A:1007504124603.

[29] Enlow EM, Luft JC, Napier ME, DeSimone JM. Potent engineered PLGA nanoparticles by virtue of exceptionally high chemotherapeutic loadings. Nano Letters. 2011;11(2): 808–813. DOI: 10.1021/nl104117p.

[30] Chaisri W, Hennink WE, Okonogi S. Preparation and characterization of cephalexin loaded PLGA microspheres. Current Drug Delivery. 2009;6(1):69–75. DOI: 10.2174/156720109787048186.

[31] Cohen-Sela E, Teitlboim S, Chorny M, Koroukhov N, Danenberg HD, Gao J, et al. Single and double emulsion manufacturing techniques of an amphiphilic drug in PLGA nanoparticles: formulations of mithramycin and bioactivity. Journal of Pharmaceutical Sciences. 2009;98(4):1452–1462. DOI: 10.1002/jps.21527.

[32] Kang F, Singh J. Effect of additives on the release of a model protein from PLGA microspheres. AAPS PharmSciTech. 2001;2(4):86–92. DOI: 10.1007/BF02830570.

[33] Dong Y, Feng S-S. Poly(D,L-lactide-co-glycolide)(PLGA) nanoparticles prepared by high pressure homogenization for paclitaxel chemotherapy. International Journal of Pharmaceutics. 2007;342(1):208–214. DOI: 10.1016/j.ijpharm.2007.04.031.

[34] Paillard-Giteau A, Tran V, Thomas O, Garric X, Coudane J, Marchal S, et al. Effect of various additives and polymers on lysozyme release from PLGA microspheres prepared by an s/o/w emulsion technique. European Journal of Pharmaceutics and Biopharmaceutics. 2010;75(2):128–136. DOI: 10.1016/j.ejpb.2010.03.005.

[35] Thevenot J, Troutier A-L, Putaux J-L, Delair T, Ladaviere C. Effect of the polymer nature on the structural organization of lipid/polymer particle assemblies. The Journal of Physical Chemistry B. 2008;112(44):13812–13822. DOI: 10.1021/jp805865r.

[36] Liao Z, Wang H, Wang X, Zhao P, Wang S, Su W, et al. Multifunctional nanoparticles composed of a poly(DL-lactide-coglycolide) core and a paramagnetic liposome shell for simultaneous magnetic resonance imaging and targeted therapeutics. Advanced Functional Materials. 2011;21(6):1179–1186. DOI: 10.1002/adfm.201002314.

[37] Wang H, Zhao P, Su W, Wang S, Liao Z, Niu R, et al. PLGA/polymeric liposome for targeted drug and gene co-delivery. Biomaterials. 2010;31(33):8741–8748. DOI: 10.1016/j.biomaterials.2010.07.082.

[38] Liang XF, Wang HJ, Luo H, Tian H, Zhang BB, Hao LJ, et al. Characterization of novel multifunctional cationic polymeric liposomes formed from octadecyl quaternized carboxymethyl chitosan/cholesterol and drug encapsulation. Langmuir. 2008;24(14):7147–7153. DOI: 10.1021/la703775a.

[39] Zhao P, Wang H, Yu M, Liao Z, Wang X, Zhang F, et al. Paclitaxel loaded folic acid targeted nanoparticles of mixed lipid-shell and polymer-core: in vitro and in vivo evaluation. European Journal of Pharmaceutics and Biopharmaceutics. 2012;81(2):248–256. DOI: 10.1016/j.ejpb.2012.03.004.

[40] Li X, Anton N, Arpagaus C, Belleteix F, Vandamme TF. Nanoparticles by spray drying using innovative new technology: the Büchi Nano Spray Dryer B-90. Journal of Controlled Release. 2010;147(2):304–310. DOI: 10.1016/j.jconrel.2010.07.113.

[41] Hitzman CJ, Elmquist WF, Wattenberg LW, Wiedmann TS. Development of a respirable, sustained release microcarrier for 5-fluorouracil I: in vitro assessment of liposomes, microspheres, and lipid coated nanoparticles. Journal of Pharmaceutical Sciences. 2006;95(5):1114–1126. DOI: 10.1002/jps.20591.

[42] Keloglu N, Verrier B, Trimaille T, Sohier J. Controlled association and delivery of nanoparticles from jet-sprayed hybrid microfibrillar matrices. Colloids and Surfaces B: Biointerfaces. 2016;140:142–149. DOI: 10.1016/j.colsurfb.2015.12.039.

[43] Hasan W, Chu K, Gullapalli A, Dunn SS, Enlow EM, Luft JC, et al. Delivery of multiple siRNAs using lipid-coated PLGA nanoparticles for treatment of prostate cancer. Nano Letters. 2011;12(1):287–292. DOI: 10.1021/nl2035354.

[44] Caldorera-Moore M, Glangchai L, Shi L, Roy K. Step and flash imprint lithography for the fabrication of shape-specific, enzymatically-triggered, drug nanocarriers. UNE. 2016;13:15.

[45] Cheow WS, Hadinoto K. Factors affecting drug encapsulation and stability of lipid–polymer hybrid nanoparticles. Colloids and Surfaces B: Biointerfaces. 2011;85(2):214–220. DOI: 10.1016/j.colsurfb.2011.02.033.

[46] D'Addio SM, Prud'homme RK. Controlling drug nanoparticle formation by rapid precipitation. Advanced Drug Delivery Reviews. 2011;63(6):417–426. DOI: 10.1016/j.addr.2011.04.005.

[47] Freese C, Gibson MI, Klok H-A, Unger RE, Kirkpatrick CJ. Size-and coating-dependent uptake of polymer-coated gold nanoparticles in primary human dermal microvascular endothelial cells. Biomacromolecules. 2012;13(5):1533–1543. DOI: 10.1021/bm300248u.

[48] Chu C-H, Wang Y-C, Huang H-Y, Wu L-C, Yang C-S. Ultrafine PEG-coated poly(lactic-co-glycolic acid) nanoparticles formulated by hydrophobic surfactant-assisted one-pot synthesis for biomedical applications. Nanotechnology. 2011;22(18):185601. DOI: 10.1088/0957-4484/22/18/185601/meta.

[49] Liu Y, Pan J, Feng S-S. Nanoparticles of lipid monolayer shell and biodegradable polymer core for controlled release of paclitaxel: effects of surfactants on particles size, characteristics and in vitro performance. International Journal of Pharmaceutics. 2010;395(1):243–250. DOI: 10.1016/j.ijpharm.2010.05.008.

[50] Bershteyn A, Chaparro J, Yau R, Kim M, Reinherz E, Ferreira-Moita L, et al. Polymer-supported lipid shells, onions, and flowers. Soft Matter. 2008;4(9):1787–1791. DOI: 10.1039/B804933E.

[51] Yang Z, Luo X, Zhang X, Liu J, Jiang Q. Targeted delivery of 10-hydroxycamptothecin to human breast cancers by cyclic RGD-modified lipid-polymer hybrid nanoparticles. Biomedical Materials. 2013;8(2):025012. DOI: 10.1088/1748-6041.

[52] Zheng M, Gong P, Zheng C, Zhao P, Luo Z, Ma Y, et al. Lipid-polymer nanoparticles for folate-receptor targeting delivery of doxorubicin. Journal of Nanoscience and Nanotechnology. 2015;15(7):4792–4798. DOI: 10.1166/jnn.2015.9604.

[53] Yang Z, Tang W, Luo X, Zhang X, Zhang C, Li H, et al. Dual-ligand modified polymer-lipid hybrid nanoparticles for docetaxel targeting delivery to Her2/neu overexpressed human breast cancer cells. Journal of Biomedical Nanotechnology. 2015;11(8):1401–1417. DOI: 10.1166/jbn.2015.2086.

[54] Shi J, Xiao Z, Votruba AR, Vilos C, Farokhzad OC. Differentially charged hollow core/shell lipid–polymer–lipid hybrid nanoparticles for small interfering RNA delivery. Angewandte Chemie. 2011;123(31):7165–7169. DOI: 10.1002/ange.201101554.

[55] Mandal B, Bhattacharjee H, Mittal N, Sah H, Balabathula P, Thoma LA, et al. Core–shell-type lipid–polymer hybrid nanoparticles as a drug delivery platform. Nanomedicine: Nanotechnology, Biology and Medicine. 2013;9(4):474–491. DOI: 10.1016/j.nano.2012.11.010.

[56] Su C-W, Chiang M-Y, Lin Y-L, Tsai N-M, Chen Y-P, Li W-M, et al. Sodium dodecyl sulfate-modified doxorubicin-loaded chitosan-lipid nanocarrier with multi polysaccharide-lecithin nanoarchitecture for augmented bioavailability and stability of oral administration in vitro and in vivo. Journal of Biomedical Nanotechnology. 2016;12(5):962–972. DOI: 10.1166/jbn.2016.2227.

[57] Su X, Fricke J, Kavanagh DG, Irvine DJ. In vitro and in vivo mRNA delivery using lipid-enveloped pH-responsive polymer nanoparticles. Molecular Pharmaceutics. 2011;8(3):774–787. DOI: 10.1021/mp100390w.

[58] Ling G, Zhang P, Zhang W, Sun J, Meng X, Qin Y, et al. Development of novel self-assembled DS-PLGA hybrid nanoparticles for improving oral bioavailability of vincristine sulfate by P-gp inhibition. Journal of Controlled Release. 2010;148(2):241–248. DOI: 10.1016/j.jconrel.2010.08.010.

[59] Zhang L, Chan JM, Gu FX, Rhee J-W, Wang AZ, Radovic-Moreno AF, et al. Self-assembled lipid–polymer hybrid nanoparticles: a robust drug delivery platform. ACS Nano. 2008;2(8):1696–1702. DOI: 10.1021/nn800275r.

[60] He C, Lu J, Lin W. Hybrid nanoparticles for combination therapy of cancer. Journal of Controlled Release. 2015;219:224–236. DOI: 10.1080/17425247.2016.1211637.

[61] Yang X-Z, Dou S, Wang Y-C, Long H-Y, Xiong M-H, Mao C-Q, et al. Single-step assembly of cationic lipid–polymer hybrid nanoparticles for systemic delivery of siRNA. ACS Nano. 2012;6(6):4955–4965. DOI: 10.1021/nn300500u.

[62] Wang G, Yu B, Wu Y, Huang B, Yuan Y, Liu CS. Controlled preparation and antitumor efficacy of vitamin E TPGS-functionalized PLGA nanoparticles for delivery of paclitaxel. International Journal of Pharmaceutics. 2013;446(1):24–33. DOI: 10.1016/j.ijpharm.2013.02.004.

[63] Fang RH, Aryal S, Hu C-MJ, Zhang L. Quick synthesis of lipid-polymer hybrid nanoparticles with low polydispersity using a single-step sonication method. Langmuir. 2010;26(22):16958–16962. DOI: 10.1021/la103576a.

[64] Liu Y, Li K, Pan J, Liu B, Feng S-S. Folic acid conjugated nanoparticles of mixed lipid monolayer shell and biodegradable polymer core for targeted delivery of Docetaxel. Biomaterials. 2010;31(2):330–338. DOI: 10.1016/j.biomaterials.2009.09.036.

[65] Mandal B, Mittal NK, Balabathula P, Thoma LA, Wood GC. Development and in vitro evaluation of core–shell type lipid–polymer hybrid nanoparticles for the delivery of erlotinib in non-small cell lung cancer. European Journal of Pharmaceutical Sciences. 2016;81:162–171. DOI: 10.1016/j.ejps.2015.10.021.

[66] Wong HL, Bendayan R, Rauth AM, Xue HY, Babakhanian K, Wu XY. A mechanistic study of enhanced doxorubicin uptake and retention in multidrug resistant breast cancer cells using a polymer-lipid hybrid nanoparticle system. Journal of Pharmacology and Experimental Therapeutics. 2006;317(3):1372–1381. DOI: 10.1124/jpet.106.101154.

[67] Wong HL, Bendayan R, Rauth AM, Wu XY. Simultaneous delivery of doxorubicin and GG918 (Elacridar) by new polymer-lipid hybrid nanoparticles (PLN) for enhanced treatment of multidrug-resistant breast cancer. Journal of Controlled Release. 2006;116 (3):275–284. DOI: 10.1016/j.jconrel.2006.09.007.

[68] Kumar S, Lather V, Pandita D. Green synthesis of therapeutic nanoparticles: an expanding horizon. Nanomedicine. 2015;10(15):2451–2471. DOI: 10.2217/nnm.15.112.

[69] Payyappilly SS, Panja S, Mandal P, Dhara S, Chattopadhyay S. Organic solvent-free low temperature method of preparation for self assembled amphiphilic poly(ϵ-caprolactone)–poly(ethylene glycol) block copolymer based nanocarriers for protein delivery. Colloids and Surfaces B: Biointerfaces. 2015;135:510–517. DOI: 10.1016/j.colsurfb.2015.07.075.

[70] Kumar S, Lather V, Pandita D. A facile green approach to prepare core-shell hybrid PLGA nanoparticles for resveratrol delivery. International Journal of Biological Macromolecules 2016;84:380–384. DOI: 10.1016/j.ijbiomac.2015.12.036.

[71] Gómez-Romero P, Sanchez C. Hybrid materials, functional applications. An introduction: Wiley-VCH Verlag GmbH & Co. KGaA: Weinheim, Germany; 2004.

[72] Van Bommel KJ, Friggeri A, Shinkai S. Organic templates for the generation of inorganic materials. Angewandte Chemie, International Edition. 2003;42(9):980–999. DOI: 10.1002/anie.200390284.

[73] Sanchez C, Belleville P, Popall M, Nicole L. Applications of advanced hybrid organic–inorganic nanomaterials: from laboratory to market. Chemical Society Reviews. 2011;40(2):696–753. DOI: 10.1039/C0CS00136H.

[74] Corriu RJ, Mehdi A, Reyé C, Thieuleux C. Control of coordination chemistry in both the framework and the pore channels of mesoporous hybrid materials. New Journal of Chemistry. 2003;27(6):905–908. DOI: 10.1039/B302027D.

[75] Shen M, Shi X. Dendrimer-based organic/inorganic hybrid nanoparticles in biomedical applications. Nanoscale. 2010;2(9):1596–1610. DOI: 10.1039/C0NR00072H.

[76] Agrawal U, Chashoo G, Sharma PR, Kumar A, Saxena AK, Vyas SP. Tailored polymer–lipid hybrid nanoparticles for the delivery of drug conjugate: dual strategy for brain targeting. Colloids and Surfaces B: Biointerfaces. 2015;126:414–425. DOI: 10.1016/j.colsurfb.2014.12.045.

[77] Carbone C, Manno D, Serra A, Musumeci T, Pepe V, Tisserand C, et al. Innovative hybrid vs polymeric nanocapsules: the influence of the cationic lipid coating on the "4S". Colloids and Surfaces B: Biointerfaces. 2016;141:450–457. DOI: 10.1016/j.colsurfb.2016.02.002.

[78] Chan JM, Zhang L, Yuet KP, Liao G, Rhee J-W, Langer R, et al. PLGA–lecithin–PEG core–shell nanoparticles for controlled drug delivery. Biomaterials. 2009;30(8):1627–1634. DOI: 10.1016/j.biomaterials.2008.12.013.

[79] Clawson C, Ton L, Aryal S, Fu V, Esener S, Zhang L. Synthesis and characterization of lipid–polymer hybrid nanoparticles with pH-triggered poly(ethylene glycol) shedding. Langmuir. 2011;27(17):10556–10561. DOI: 10.1021/la202123e.

[80] Troutier A-L, Delair T, Pichot C, Ladavière C. Physicochemical and interfacial investigation of lipid/polymer particle assemblies. Langmuir. 2005;21(4):1305–1313. DOI: 10.1021/la047659t.

[81] Devrim B, Kara A, Vural I, Bozkir A. Lysozyme-loaded lipid-polymer hybrid nanoparticles: preparation, characterization and colloidal stability evaluation. Drug Development and Industrial Pharmacy. 2016:1–12. DOI: 10.1080/03639045.2016.1180392.

[82] Dim N, Perepelyuk M, Gomes O, Thangavel C, Liu Y, Den R, et al. Novel targeted siRNA-loaded hybrid nanoparticles: preparation, characterization and in vitro evaluation. Journal of Nanobiotechnology. 2015;13:61. DOI: 10.1186/s12951-015-0124-2.

[83] El-Sherbiny IM, El-Shibiny A, Salih E. Photo-induced green synthesis and antimicrobial efficacy of poly (ε-caprolactone)/curcumin/grape leaf extract-silver hybrid nanoparticles. Journal of Photochemistry and Photobiology B: Biology. 2016;160:355–363.

[84] Wong HL, Rauth AM, Bendayan R, Manias JL, Ramaswamy M, Liu Z, et al. A new polymer–lipid hybrid nanoparticle system increases cytotoxicity of doxorubicin against multidrug-resistant human breast cancer cells. Pharmaceutical Research. 2006;23(7):1574–1585. DOI: 10.1007/s11095-006-0282-x.

[85] Xie Y, Qiao H, Su Z, Chen M, Ping Q, Sun M. PEGylated carboxymethyl chitosan/calcium phosphate hybrid anionic nanoparticles mediated hTERT siRNA delivery for anticancer therapy. Biomaterials. 2014;35(27):7978–7991. DOI: 10.1016/j.biomaterials.2014.05.068.

[86] Zhang J, Hu J, Chan HF, Skibba M, Liang G, Chen M. iRGD decorated lipid-polymer hybrid nanoparticles for targeted co-delivery of doxorubicin and sorafenib to enhance anti-hepatocellular carcinoma efficacy. Nanomedicine. 2016;12(5):1303–1311. DOI: 10.1016/j.nano.2016.01.017.

[87] Zhang RX, Cai P, Zhang T, Chen K, Li J, Cheng J, et al. Polymer–lipid hybrid nanoparticles synchronize pharmacokinetics of co-encapsulated doxorubicin–mitomycin C and enable their spatiotemporal co-delivery and local bioavailability in breast tumor. Nanomedicine: Nanotechnology, Biology and Medicine 2016;12(5):1279–1290. DOI: 10.1016/j.nano.2015.12.383.

[88] Kandel PK, Fernando LP, Ackroyd PC, Christensen KA. Incorporating functionalized polyethylene glycol lipids into reprecipitated conjugated polymer nanoparticles for bioconjugation and targeted labeling of cells. Nanoscale. 2011;3(3):1037–1045. DOI: 10.1039/C0NR00746C.

[89] Sengupta S, Eavarone D, Capila I, Zhao G, Watson N, Kiziltepe T, et al. Temporal targeting of tumour cells and neovasculature with a nanoscale delivery system. Nature. 2005;436(7050):568–572. DOI: 10.1038/nature03794.

[90] Palange AL, Di Mascolo D, Carallo C, Gnasso A, Decuzzi P. Lipid–polymer nanoparticles encapsulating curcumin for modulating the vascular deposition of breast cancer cells. Nanomedicine: Nanotechnology, Biology and Medicine. 2014;10(5):e991-e1002. DOI: 10.1016/j.nano.2014.02.004.

[91] Wang W, Chen S, Zhang L, Wu X, Wang J, Chen J-F, et al. Poly(lactic acid)/chitosan hybrid nanoparticles for controlled release of anticancer drug. Materials Science and Engineering C 2015;46:514–520. DOI: 10.1016/j.msec.2014.10.048.

[92] Yan J, Wang Y, Zhang X, Liu S, Tian C, Wang H. Targeted nanomedicine for prostate cancer therapy: docetaxel and curcumin co-encapsulated lipid-polymer hybrid nanoparticles for the enhanced anti-tumor activity in vitro and in vivo. Drug Delivery. 2016;23(5):1757–1762. DOI: 10.3109/10717544.2015.1069423.

[93] Shi K, Zhou J, Zhang Q, Gao H, Liu Y, Zong T, et al. Arginine-glycine-aspartic acid-modified lipid-polymer hybrid nanoparticles for docetaxel delivery in glioblastoma multiforme. Journal of Biomedical Nanotechnology. 2015;11(3):382–391. DOI: 10.1166/jbn.2015.1965.

[94] Ramasamy T, Tran TH, Choi JY, Cho HJ, Kim JH, Yong CS, et al. Layer-by-layer coated lipid–polymer hybrid nanoparticles designed for use in anticancer drug delivery. Carbohydrate Polymers. 2014;102:653–661. DOI: 10.1016/j.carbpol.2013.11.009.

[95] Wu B, Yu P, Cui C, Wu M, Zhang Y, Liu L, et al. Folate-containing reduction-sensitive lipid-polymer hybrid nanoparticles for targeted delivery of doxorubicin. Biomaterials Science. 2015;3(4):655–664. DOI: 10.1039/C4BM00462K.

[96] Messerschmidt SK, Musyanovych A, Altvater M, Scheurich P, Pfizenmaier K, Landfester K, et al. Targeted lipid-coated nanoparticles: delivery of tumor necrosis factor-functionalized particles to tumor cells. Journal of Controlled Release. 2009;137(1):69–77. DOI: 10.1016/j.jconrel.2009.03.010.

[97] Varthya M, Pawar H, Singh C, Dora CP, Jena SK, Suresh S. Development of novel polymer-lipid hybrid nanoparticles of tamoxifen: in vitro and in vivo evaluation. Journal of Nanoscience and Nanotechnology. 2016;16(1):253–260. DOI: 10.1166/jnn.2016.10651.

[98] Kumar S, Sangwan P, Lather V, Pandita D. Biocompatible PLGA-oil hybrid nanoparticles for high loading and controlled delivery of resveratrol. Journal of Drug Delivery Science and Technology. 2015;30:54–62. DOI: 10.1016/j.jddst.2015.09.016.

[99] Makino K, Yamada T, Kimura M, Oka T, Ohshima H, Kondo T. Temperature-and ionic strength-induced conformational changes in the lipid head group region of liposomes as suggested by zeta potential data. Biophysical Chemistry. 1991;41(2):175–183. DOI: 10.1016/0301-4622(91)80017-L.

[100] Hallan SS, Kaur P, Kaur V, Mishra N, Vaidya B. Lipid polymer hybrid as emerging tool in nanocarriers for oral drug delivery. Artificial Cells, Nanomedicine, and Biotechnology. 2016;44(1):334–349. DOI: 10.3109/21691401.2014.951721.

[101] Mornet S, Lambert O, Duguet E, Brisson A. The formation of supported lipid bilayers on silica nanoparticles revealed by cryoelectron microscopy. Nano Letters. 2005;5(2): 281–285. DOI: 10.1021/nl048153y.

[102] Schmitt J, Danner B, Bayerl TM. Polymer cushions in supported phospholipid bilayers reduce significantly the frictional drag between bilayer and solid surface. Langmuir. 2001;17(1):244–246. DOI: 10.1021/la001275v.

[103] Romberg B, Hennink WE, Storm G. Sheddable coatings for long-circulating nanoparticles. Pharmaceutical Research. 2008;25(1):55–71. DOI: 10.1007/s11095-007-9348-7.

[104] Zhong Q, Chinta DMD, Pamujula S, Wang H, Yao X, Mandal TK, et al. Optimization of DNA delivery by three classes of hybrid nanoparticle/DNA complexes. Journal of Nanobiotechnology. 2010;8(1):1. DOI: 10.1186/1477-3155-8-6.

[105] Bershteyn A, Hanson MC, Crespo MP, Moon JJ, Li AV, Suh H, et al. Robust IgG responses to nanograms of antigen using a biomimetic lipid-coated particle vaccine. Journal of Controlled Release. 2012;157(3):354–365. DOI: 10.1016/j.jconrel.2011.07.029.

[106] Luo Y, Teng Z, Li Y, Wang Q. Solid lipid nanoparticles for oral drug delivery: chitosan coating improves stability, controlled delivery, mucoadhesion and cellular uptake. Carbohydrate Polymers. 2015;122:221–229. DOI: 10.1016/j.carbpol.2014.12.084.

[107] Harde H, Agrawal AK, Jain S. Tetanus toxoids loaded glucomannosylated chitosan based nanohoming vaccine adjuvant with improved oral stability and immunostimulatory response. Pharmaceutical Research. 2015;32(1):122–134. DOI: 10.1007/s11095-014-1449-5.

[108] Badhulika S, Terse-Thakoor T, Villarreal C, Mulchandani A. Graphene hybrids: synthesis strategies and applications in sensors and sensitized solar cells. Frontiers in Chemistry. 2015;3. DOI: 10.3389/fchem.2015.00038.

[109] Rehman M, Asadullah Madni AI, Khan WS, Khan MI, Mahmood MA, Ashfaq M, et al. Solid and liquid lipid-based binary solid lipid nanoparticles of diacerein: in vitro evaluation of sustained release, simultaneous loading of gold nanoparticles, and potential thermoresponsive behavior. International Journal of Nanomedicine. 2015;10:2805. DOI: 10.2147/IJN.S67147.

[110] Javed I, Hussain SZ, Shahzad A, Khan JM, Rehman M, Usman F, et al. Lecithin-gold hybrid nanocarriers as efficient and pH selective vehicles for oral delivery of diacerein—in-vitro and in-vivo study. Colloids and Surfaces B: Biointerfaces. 2016; 141:1–9. DOI: 10.1016/j.colsurfb.2016.01.022.

[111] Umair M, Javed I, Rehman M, Madni A, Javeed A, Ghafoor A, et al. Nanotoxicity of inert materials: the case of gold, silver and iron. Journal of Pharmacy & Pharmaceutical Sciences. 2016;19(2):161–180. DOI: 10.18433/J31021.

[112] McCarthy JR, Weissleder R. Multifunctional magnetic nanoparticles for targeted imaging and therapy. Advanced Drug Delivery Reviews. 2008;60(11):1241–1251. DOI: 10.1016/j.addr.2008.03.014.

[113] Lee N, Yoo D, Ling D, Cho MH, Hyeon T, Cheon J. Iron oxide based nanoparticles for multimodal imaging and magnetoresponsive therapy. Chemical Reviews. 2015;115(19):10637–10689. DOI: 10.1021/acs.chemrev.5b00112.

[114] Shi J, Jiang Y, Wang X, Wu H, Yang D, Pan F, et al. Design and synthesis of organic–inorganic hybrid capsules for biotechnological applications. Chemical Society Reviews. 2014;43(15):5192–5210. DOI: 10.1039/C4CS00108G.

[115] Portney NG, Singh K, Chaudhary S, Destito G, Schneemann A, Manchester M, et al. Organic and inorganic nanoparticle hybrids. Langmuir. 2005;21(6):2098–2103. DOI: 10.1021/la047525f.

[116] Zhou W, Huang P-JJ, Ding J, Liu J. Aptamer-based biosensors for biomedical diagnostics. Analyst. 2014;139(11):2627–2640. DOI: 10.1039/C4AN00132J.

[117] Sreejith S, Ma X, Zhao Y. Graphene oxide wrapping on squaraine-loaded mesoporous silica nanoparticles for bioimaging. Journal of the American Chemical Society. 2012;134(42):17346–17349. DOI: 10.1021/ja305352d.

[118] Maji SK, Mandal AK, Nguyen KT, Borah P, Zhao Y. Cancer cell detection and therapeutics using peroxidase-active nanohybrid of gold nanoparticle-loaded mesoporous silica-coated graphene. ACS Applied Materials & Interfaces. 2015;7(18):9807–9816. DOI: 10.1021/acsami.5b01758.

Chapter 5

Numerical Simulation and Experimental Testing to Improve Olfactory Drug Delivery with Electric Field Guidance of Charged Particles

Jinxiang Xi and Xiuhua April Si

Additional information is available at the end of the chapter

http://dx.doi.org/ 10.5772/65858

Abstract

Even though the direct nose-to-brain drug delivery has many clinical benefits, there are limited successes in delivering medication aerosols to the olfactory mucosa with standard inhalation devices. In this study, different delivery techniques were assessed in terms of their capacities to deliver drug aerosols to the olfactory epithelium. Specifically, the feasibility of electric field guidance of charged aerosols to the olfactory mucosa was evaluated in an image-based nose model both numerically and experimentally. Multi-sectional nasal cast replicas were fabricated using a 3-D printer to measure the olfactory deposition rates and visualize the deposition distributions. An intranasal deposition test platform was developed that comprised an electric field guidance system, a dry powder charging device, and a point-release nozzle. Numerical simulations were conducted using both ANSYS Fluent and COMSOL. We demonstrated that it is feasible to control charged particles inside the human nose use an external electric field. Both the point-release technique and electric field guidance of drug particles are essential in attaining optimal olfactory doses. Consistent deposition patterns were achieved between in vitro experiments and computational simulations. Future investigations are warrnated for further improvements of olfactory delivery through refining the particle generation, charging, and releasing, and navigation systems.

Keywords: intranasal drug delivery, olfactory region, particle point release, electric field guidance, charged particles, nose-to-brain drug delivery

1. Introduction

Drug delivery for treating neurological disorders such as brain tumors is often forestalled by the blood-brain-barrier (BBB), a network of endothelial cells with tight junctions in the brain's capillaries. The BBB, which can effectively protect the central nervous system (CNS) from pathogens, also prevents therapeutically agents from the diseased tissues in the CNS [1]. For years, the BBB has thwarted the utilizations of many new neurological medications for the treatment of CNS diseases such as brain tumors, depression, and Alzheimer's disease [2, 3].

Intranasal drug delivery to the olfactory epithelium is a noninvasive technique in which medications can bypass the BBB and enter the brain, eliciting a quick uptake and action onset of the therapeutic agents [3, 4]. However, there are many challenges that preclude effective drug delivery to the olfactory region. Very low doses can be delivered to the olfactory region (<1%) via the nasal route using standard nasal devices such as nasal pumps and sprays [5, 6]. It is primarily due to the complicated structure of the human nose, which is composed of convoluted, narrow, and passages. The olfactory mucosa is located at the uppermost part of the nose and is poorly ventilated due to its secluded location [7, 8]. As a result, standard nasal devices have limited success in olfactory drug delivery in that they rely on aerodynamic forces or particle inertia to drive medications to the target area [9]. After administration, particles travel passively with the nasal airflow. Thus, the behavior and fate of these aerosols are primarily dependent on their release positions and initial speeds. Due to the complex nasal structure, most of the medications will be trapped by the nasal valve and turbinate, with very few left that can make their final journey to the olfactory mucosa [10].

Nasal deposition of inhaled aerosols in humans has been extensively investigated both experimentally and numerically. Despite the high variability among subjects, these studies have persistently demonstrated that intranasal drug delivery can be influenced by multiple factors, including patient breathing, nasal devices, administration technique, and drug formulation. Furthermore, local or cellular-level deposition has been shown to be a more appropriate parameter than the total deposition in predicting adverse health effects or therapeutic outcomes. However, reports of local doses are still rare in comparison with extensive reports of total deposition fractions in the literature.

New techniques have been under active investigation to improve the olfactory delivery efficiency. Wang et al. [11] proposed to insert a catheter into the nose and administer drugs beneath the olfactory region. However, due to its invasive nature, this method has the risk to damage the wall tissues when guiding the catheter to the olfactory proximity, and patient compliance is expected to be low. Gizurarson [12] tested a nozzle with a narrow spray angle in hope that aerosols can penetrate into the posterior nose and the olfactory mucosa. A high pressure was necessary for this technique to overcome the nasal resistance so that particles can penetrate into the superior meatus. Hoekman and Ho [13] proposed to use a swirling flow in additional to the narrow spray plume so that particles can penetrate deeper into the upper posterior nose. Persistent higher doses in the olfactory region with swirling flows were measured in rats relative to nonswirling flows. However, extrapolating rat data to humans is difficult because of large interspecies discrepancies [14]. For instance, the olfactory region of a Sprague-Dawley rat covers 45% of the nasal surface, while only 5.2% of the human nasal surface is lined by the olfactory epitheliums in humans [15]. Realizing that a particle released into the nostril at a different location will follow a specific path, Si et al. [6] release drug particles from a selected site in the nostril (termed as point release). Improved dosage in the olfactory region was demonstrated using the point releasing than the traditional whole nostril releasing; however, the improvements are limited and still fall short of the doses to be clinically significant. Considering all the techniques aforementioned, it is noticed that once the particles are released into the nose the particle motions are dictated solely by the aerodynamic force. Due to the complex structure of the nasal structure, most particles will deposit in the nasal valve and turbinate region and only a low percentage of particles penetrate into the olfactory region.

Previous studies have suggested that charged particles under an appropriate electric field can improve nasal and pulmonary drug deliveries [16–18]. Improved dosing of charged particles has been demonstrated in the respiratory tract of both humans and animals [19–29]. Noticing that low olfactory deposition mainly result from the lack of control over particle dynamics in the nose, Xi et al. [25] numerically investigated the transport and deposition of charged particles under different electric strengths and showed that significantly enhanced olfactory dosage is practical by optimizing the electric field strength and particle releasing locations. Similarly, enhanced olfactory dosing can also be attained by using magnetic control of ferromagnetic particles. Preliminary computational simulations predicted a 45.0% deposition fraction for ferromagnetic particles, and the optimal particle diameter is around 15 μm [25].

One issue of intranasal drug delivery of nebulized droplets or small particles is the unwanted dosages into the lungs. One strategy to address this issue is the bi-directional delivery method, which administers medications into one nostril when the patient blows into the apparatus [30]. This method takes advantage of the nature that the soft palate lifts up during exhalation through the mouth, which closes the oropharynx and separates the nasal cavity from the rest of the respiratory tract. As a result, particle penetration into the lungs can be avoided. Moreover, the particles enter one nostril and exit from the other, which allows an increased time for drug deposition. This method did show an increase in medications depositing in the nasal cavity but failed to provide a practical way of dispensing an appreciable amount of medications to the olfactory region [31, 32]. It is hypothesized that by combining the electric guidance of charged particles with the bi-directional strategy, the olfactory dosage can be further enhanced.

The objective of this chapter is to improve the targeted delivery of neurological medications to the olfactory region using both computational modeling and *in vitro* experiments in an image-based nasal airway model. Different strategies were explored to control the intranasal particle motions in order to maximize the dose to the olfactory region and minimize the drug losses in other regions. These strategies include point release, vestibular intubation, deep intubation, and electric guidance of charged particles. Effect of breathing conditions, such as normal inhalation and bi-directional breathing, was also considered.

2. Design of experiments

2.1. Image-based reconstruction of nasal airway model

First, building anatomically accurate airway models is crucial for the assessment of the health outcomes of inhalation therapies. **Figure 1** illustrates the procedures of the translation from medical images into a high-quality computational mesh or *in vitro* casts of the nose-pharynx. To reconstruct the 3-D nasal airway model, MRI scans (512 × 512 pixel resolution) of a healthy 53-year-old male were used. The multislice MRI images were segmented using MIMICS (Materialise, Ann Arbor, MI) to convert the raw image data into a set of cross-sectional contours that define the solid geometry (**Figure 1a**). A surface geometry was reconstructed based on these contours in Gambit (Ansys, Inc.). This surface geometry as shown in **Figure 1b** was subsequently imported into ANSYS ICEM (Ansys, Inc.) for meshing. In general, unless for extremely high-quality image data, a solid model that is directly reconstructed from medical images cannot be used for computational meshing due to the artifacts and resolution limits inherent in current imaging techniques. Considering the high complexity of the nasal airway structure, an unstructured mesh was generated with fine boy-fitted cells in the near-wall region (**Figure 1c**). This nasal geometry has been reconstructed with minimal surface smoothing and was intended to accurately represent the nasal anatomy of human adults. More details of image-based model development can be viewed in a recent video article from our group [33]. This model was also manufactured into hollow casts for *in vitro* studies using 3-D prototyping techniques (**Figure 1d**).

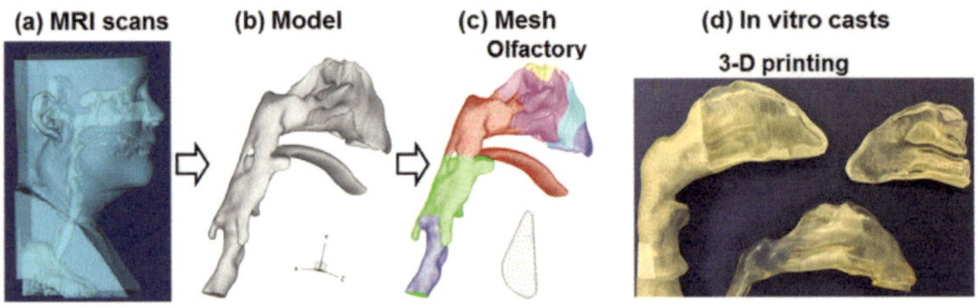

Figure 1. Procedures of translating medical images into computational mesh and *in vitro* casts. First, MRI scans were segmented to reconstruct the airway surface model. Second, high-quality computational mesh was generated with fine near-wall cells. Hollow *in vitro* cast replicas were also fabricated using 3-D printing technique and were used for experimental deposition studies. In order to study deposition distributions, the nasal cavity was divided into different regions: vestibule-valve region (VV), turbinate region (TR), nasopharynx (NP), and olfactory region (OL) that was at the very top of the nasal cavity (yellow color in middle panel).

2.2. Computational fluid-particle transport models

2.2.1. *Airflow and particle dynamics*

Depending on breathing activities, multiple flow regimes, such as laminar, transitional, or fully turbulent, can exist in the human respiratory tract. The two-order turbulence models have been shown to adequately capture the main flow features and particle transport if a fine body-fitted mesh is used near the wall [34]. In particular, the low Reynolds number (LRN) *k-ω* model has been widely adopted in computational studies of respiratory flows. It has been validated in many studies to be able to accurately predict the particle transport and deposition in the oral airway [35, 36], nasal cavity [8], and lungs [37, 38]. Moreover, the LRN *k-ω* model was demonstrated to accurately predict the flow regime transition when the turbulent viscosity approaches zero [39]. Governing equations for the turbulent kinetic energy (*k*) and dissipation rate (*ω*) can be found in Wilcox [39].

Transport of monodisperse aerosols was solved using the discrete Lagrangian tracking algorithm through the integration of the particle dynamic equation. Spherical shape was assumed for each particle. The particle diameters range from 0.2 to 5 μm, which have very low Stokes numbers ($St_k = \rho_p d_p^2 U C_c / 18\mu D_h \ll 1$), with ρ_p being the density of the particles (1.0 g/cm^3), U being the fluid velocity, C_c being the Cunningham slip factor [40], and D_h being the nostril effective diameter. The governing equation of Lagrangian tracking is

$$\frac{dv_i}{dt} = \frac{f}{\tau_p C_c}(u_i - v_i) + g_i(1-\alpha) + f_{i,Brownian} + f_{i,lift} + f_{i,electric} \tag{1}$$

where u_i is the airflow velocity, v_i is the particle speed, f is the drag coefficient, and $\tau_p = \rho_p d_p^2/18\mu$ is the particle characteristic time to respond to flow variations. The drag coefficient f was based on the equation of Morsi and Alexander [41]. Gravity and Saffman lift force were also included for particles >1 μm [42]. Brownian motion effects were included for submicron particles [35]. It was assumed that particle motion had no effect on the flow field, i.e., a one-way coupling between fluid and aerosols in light of the dilute concentration of pharmaceutical aerosols. The impact of the anisotropic flow fluctuations near the wall was also included by applying an anisotropic turbulence model as described by Matida et al. [43]:

$$u'_n = f_v \xi \sqrt{2k/3} \quad \text{and} \quad f_v = 1 - exp(-0.002y^+) \tag{2}$$

In the above equation, f_v is a damping component normal to the airway wall and ξ is a random number generated by the Gaussian probability density function.

2.2.2. *Electric field and electric force*

For the direct current (DC) field, the electric potential, U_{DC}, is attained by solving the Poisson's equation,

$$-\nabla \cdot \varepsilon_0 \varepsilon_r \nabla U = 0 \tag{3}$$

where ε_0 and ε_r are the absolute (F/m) and (dimensionless) permittivity of the free space, respectively. The zero value on the right-hand side of the equation means no space charge. For the alternating current (AC) field, the AC potential is computed by solving the conservation of electric currents [44]:

$$-\nabla \cdot \left(\sigma + j\omega\varepsilon_0\varepsilon_r\right)\nabla V = 0 \tag{4}$$

In the above equation, σ is the electrical conductivity and ω is the alternating frequency (Hz). Considering that the equations for both DC and AC fields are linear, the total electric field can be obtained by superposing the DC and AC fields.

The electric force as a function of the electric field can be expressed as

$$f_{i,electrophoretic} = neE = ne\left(E_{DC} + E_{AC}\right) \tag{5}$$

where n is the nondimensional charge number and e is the elementary charge (e = 1.6 × 10^{-19} C). E_{DC} and E_{AC} are the intensity of the DC and AC electric fields, respectively, which are calculated as follows:

$$E_{DC} = -\nabla U;\ E_{AC} = -real[\nabla \tilde{V} e^{(j\omega t)}] \tag{6}$$

The symbol $\tilde{V}$ means that the AC potential is a complex variable.

2.2.3. *Numerical methods*

To solve the concomitant flow-electric-particle multiphysics involved in each of the cases considered, ANSYS Fluent (Canonsburg, PA) and COMSOL (Burlington, MA) were employed to simulate the airflow, electric field, and particle tracing. User-supplied functions (UDFs) in the language of Fortran ad C were developed for the calculation of mass flux to the wall, initial particle profile, Brownian force [45], near-wall velocity interpolation [36], and anisotropic turbulence effect [43]. Body-fitted computational mesh was generated to resolve the large gradients of flow velocities near the airway surface. Local mesh refinement was made considering the complex anatomy of the nasal cavity. A grid independence study was performed by evaluating various grid densities, such as 0.4, 0.8, 1.2, and 2.2 million computational cells. The variation in predicted deposition fraction was 1% or less when changing the grid density from 1.2 to 2.4 million. Therefore, the computational mesh of 1.2 million cells was implemented for all subsequent simulations.

2.3. Experimental setup and materials

2.3.1. *In vitro test platform*

The *in vitro* test platform for intranasal delivery of charged particles has four components: a particle charging apparatus (**Figure 2a**), a three-dimensional replica of a normal human nasal cavity, voltage supplies to induce electric fields, and a scale to quantify deposition. A powder coating system (Powder System Solutions, Nolensville, TN) was modified to charge the dry powders. Copper plates and DC power supplies (MPJA, Lake Park, FL) were implemented to produce external electric fields. A high-precision electronic scale (Sartorius) was utilized to quantify the deposited mass of aerosols. A microscope (AmScope B120C-E1) was used to estimate the diameter of the charged particles. Details of the sectional nasal cast preparation and experimental procedures are described below.

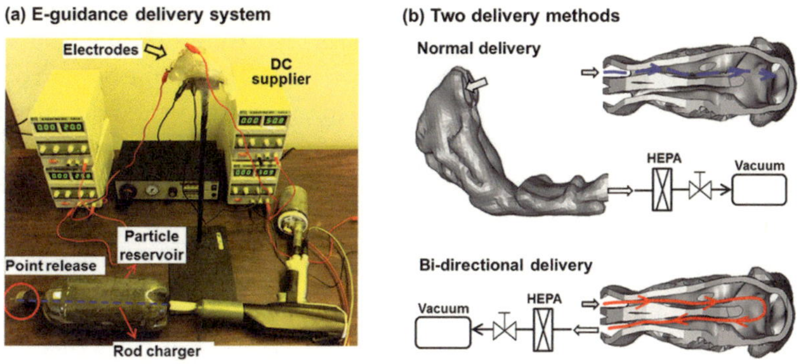

Figure 2. *In vitro* experiments to test the feasibility of electric-guided olfactory drug delivery: (a) experimental setup and (b) two delivery strategies: normal and bi-directional. In both delivery strategies, drug particles are administered into the right-side nostril. However, particles exit the airway through the trachea in the normal delivery and exit through the left nostril in the bi-directional delivery.

2.3.2. Multisectional nasal cast

A multisectional nasal replica was prepared that allows quantitative measurement of regional deposition as well as direct visualization of deposition distributions. After developing the nasal airway geometry model as listed in 2.1, Magics (Materialise, Ann Arbor, MI) was utilized to create the nasal cast wall with a constant layer of 4 mm. The nasal replica was divided into several parts: the nasal vestibule and valve, turbinate, and nasopharynx, as shown in **Figure 1b**. Step-shaped grooves were created at the ends of each replica section for proper sealing and easy assembly. To visualize deposition distributions within the nasal cavity, the nasal replica was cut open along the top ridge of the right nasal passage to disclose the septum and turbinate in the right nose. In order to characterize the olfactory doses, the section representing the olfactory mucosa was separated from the other region. An in-house 3-D printer with a resolution of 16 μm (0.0006 in) (Stratasys Objet30 Pro, Northville, MI) was utilized to fabricate the nasal casts using polypropylene (Veroclear, Northville, MI) that has a clear color and allows for a smooth surface.

2.3.3. Experimental procedures

Dry powders of 30 μm in size (matte black powder coat paint) were selected in this study for their easy availability and excellent charging properties. and easy ava. The modification made to the powder coating system integrated a charging reservoir (a 2-L bottle) to the nozzle of the charging gun (**Figure 2a**). An additional metal wire was added to extend the charging rod to the reservoir exit, with the wire's length being parallel with the direction of the flow of solid particles. A high voltage supply (Spectracoat coating system), which has an adjustable potential output of 0–100 kV, was connected to the rod. The solid particles were distributed out of a 4-mm-diameter nozzle and subsequently distributed into a multisectional nasal cast replica. Three copper-plated electrodes (A, B, C) were attached to the top of the nose replica, and one copper-plated electrode (D) was attached to the bottom of the replica. Charged dry powders were distributed from the powder coat gun for 20 seconds per trial. For the normal delivery, particles were administered into one nostril and exited through the nasopharynx (**Figure 2b**, upper panel). In contrast, for the bi-directional delivery, the bottom of the pharynx was blocked to simulate the uplifted soft palate, while particles were administered into one nostril and exited through the other (**Figure 2b**, lower panel). A vacuum pump (Robinair 3 CFM, Warren, MI) was connected to the exit of the nasal replica in each test case to simulate the respiration. An in-line flow meter (Omega, FL-510, Stamford, CT) was used to monitor the volumetric flow rate.

2.3.4. Statistical analysis

The variable of interest in this study was the ratio of the olfactory dosage to the vestibule-turbinate dosage (i.e., olfactory-nasal dosage ratio). Results were represented as the main ± standard deviation (SD), with SD being calculated from five trials for each scenario. Statistical analysis software Minitab (State College, PA) was applied to analyze the deposition data. Tukey's method and analysis of variance (ANOVA) were implemented to assess the data variances. The difference was considered statistically significant if the p-value was <0.05.

3. Results

3.1. Numerical (ANSYS Fluent) assessment of olfactory delivery with nasal intubations

Figure 3a shows the motion of 1 μm particles inside the nasal airway predicted using ANSYS Fluent. It is observed that particles that are released from the tip of the nostril move along the upper nasal cavity, while particles from the base of the nostril move along the nasal floor. At an inhalation rate of 20 L/min (normal breathing condition), it takes around 0.02–0.03 seconds for the particles to be delivered to the olfactory region after administration (**Figure 3a**). Faster movements of particles are noted in the middle passages and slow-moving aerosols are observed in the near-wall region. The numerical model in this study had been validated by comparing to *in vitro* deposition data measured in a comparable nasal replica. Good agreement was obtained between the numerically predicted and *in vitro* measurements in comparable nasal casts by Cheng et al. [46, 47] (**Figure 3b**). It is emphasized that the computational nasal airway model in this study and the *in vitro* nasal casts in Cheng et al. [46] were reconstructed from the same set of MRI images.

http://dx.doi.org/ 10.5772/65858

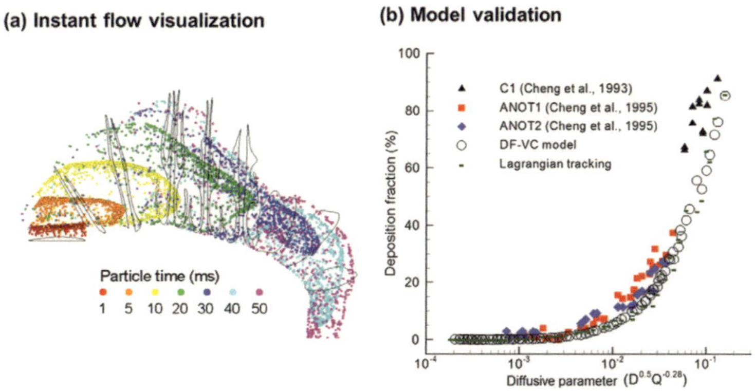

Figure 3. Nasal particle motion and model validation. (a) Snapshots of particle motion at varying instants. (b) Good agreement in nasal deposition between the numerical predictions and experimental measurements of Cheng et al. [46, 47].

In this study, we first tested the feasibility of optimizing particle release positions (smart delivery concept) for intranasal olfactory drug delivery. Two protocols were tested, with the first termed as "vestibular intubation" where particles are released from a selective point in the vestibule (**Figure 4a**), while the second protocol being the "deep intubation" with the nebulizer nozzle inserted directly below the olfactory mucosa (**Figure 4a**). In principle, particles released into the upper vestibule moves along the upper nasal passage and therefore are more likely to deposit in the olfactory region. The computational simulations also confirm that it can deliver higher doses to the olfactory region for both particle sizes considered (150 nm and 1 μm). Furthermore, the deposition pattern appears to be focused close to the olfactory region. Considering the deep intubation protocol, the nozzle was inserted right below the olfactory mucosa so that filtration by the nasal valve and turbinate can be avoided. Therefore, elevated doses were predicted in the olfactory proximity with nonsignificant doses in the middle and inferior turbinate regions.

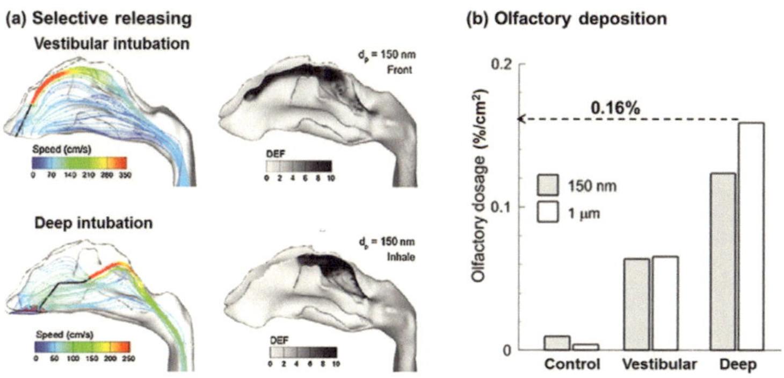

Figure 4. Two delivery protocols with selective particle releasing: vestibular intubation and deep intubation. (a) Streamlines and surface deposition. (b) Olfactory deposition rate with the vestibular and deep intubations in comparison to the conventional delivery method, which releases drugs to the entire nostril (control case).

The olfactory doses between the vestibular and deep intubation protocols, as well as the conventional delivery method, were compared on the basis of deposition fraction per area (%/cm^2) (**Figure 4b**). The surface area of the olfactory mucosa in this study (**Figure 1c**) is 6.8 cm^2. Overall speaking, both intubation protocols significantly enhanced the olfactory targeting while the deep intubation outperformed the vestibular intubation. However, it is noted that even using the deep intubation method, very low fractions of administered dose (0.16%/cm^2 or 1.09% in the olfactory region) were delivered to target, while nearly 99% was lost in other regions, causing tremendous waste and potentially significant unwanted side effects. Therefore, further efforts are needed to explore strategies that can precisely target drug particles to the olfactory region while minimizing drug loss to other tissues.

3.2. Sar-Gel visualization of nasal deposition distributions

Sar-Gel visualization of the local deposition inside the nasal replica is displayed in **Figure 5** for two common nasal spray products (Astelin and Nasonex). The angle of the spray plume was approximately 35° ± 0.8° for Astelin and 20° ± 0.5° for Nasonex. The majority of spray droplets were trapped by the narrow flow-limiting nasal valve. It is noted that the drug distribution is largely dictated by the physical properties of spray droplets. The high filtration by the slit-shaped nasal valve can be attributed to the high inertia of spray droplets that have large sizes (70–90 μm) and exit from the spray pumps with relatively high speeds. Dripping was absent in Astelin that had a wide spray plume angle, while dripping was observed in Nasonex that had a narrow plume and was prone to cause local droplet accumulation (**Figure 5a** vs. **5b**). Deposition of Astelin appeared to be more dispersed than Nasonex.

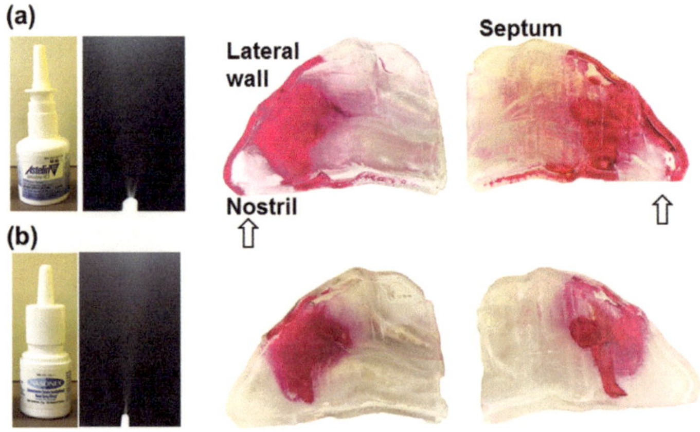

Figure 5. Deposition pattern in the nose with two nasal spray products: (a) Astelin and (b) Nasonex. The majority of spray droplets deposit in the nasal vestibule and valve region and cannot reach the olfactory region.

A commercially available jet nebulizer (Philips Respironics InnoSpire) was utilized to evaluate particle deposition in the nose. Nebulized aerosols were released into the nostril at an orientation 15° from the vertical direction. As shown in **Figure 6**, most administered droplets deposited in the anterior nose (vestibule and valve regions). Aerosol deposition in the middle and inferior turbinate was also observed, but at a lower level than the anterior nose. Almost no aerosol deposited in the superior meatus and olfactory region (dashed blue ellipse). The above deposition distribution is similar as that reported in Laube [48] who observed predominant doses in the anterior nose. Both **Figures 5** and **6** corroborate the observation that conventional nasal devices cannot deliver adequate doses to the olfactory mucosa, and thus advanced drug delivery systems are warranted in order to achieve clinical significant olfactory delivery.

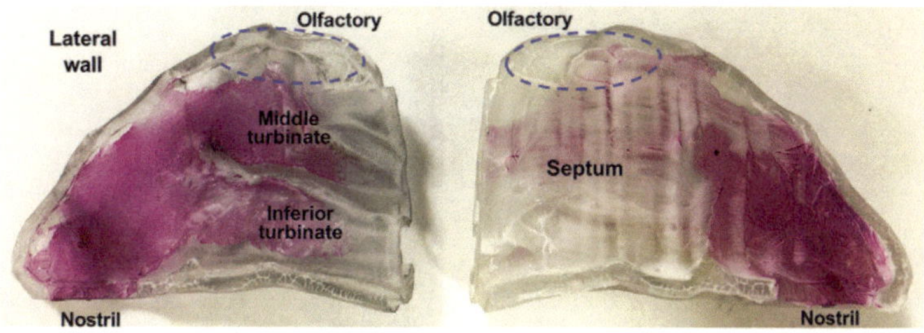

Figure 6. Sar-Gel visualization of the nasal deposition pattern using a standard nebulizer. Even though some nebulized aerosols escape the nasal valve filtration, most of them deposit in the turbinate region and only a very small fraction reaches the olfactory region.

3.3. Multiphysics (COMOL) simulations of olfactory dosing delivery of charged particles

3.3.1. Electric-guided olfactory delivery diagram

The principle of olfactory drug delivery under electric guidance is illustrated in **Figure 7**. There are four essential functions in this device: (1) generation, (2) charging, (3) focusing, and (4) navigation of the pharmaceutical aerosols (**Figure 7a**). A head brace can be added to fix the device relative to the patient's head. Commercially available nebulizers (droplets) and dry powder inhalers can be used to generate aerosolized particles [49]. Particle charging was achieved by letting particles going through a charging chamber, and the acquired charge number can be controlled by varying the voltage supply to the charging chamber [50]. The focusing chamber is composed of several slits [51], with the first slit having a positive voltage and the last one having zero voltage. When the positively charged dry powders travel through these slits, a repulsive force from the slit pushes the dry powders inward to form a focused beam; simultaneously, the forward component of the repulsion accelerates the aerosol beam to a certain exiting velocity. The benefit of knowing the initial speed of particles is that the deposition pattern can be estimated beforehand so that the optimal delivery protocol can be selected. Another benefit is that drug delivery will be more independent of the breathing condition if the initial particle velocities are much higher than the respiratory airflow velocities. This feature is very desirable for inhalation therapy for seniors or people with breathing problems or low compliance capability. After particles were administered into the nose, they will experience an external electric force and divert from their original course. For optimal drug delivery to the olfactory region, particles should move along the middle passage of the nose to minimize wall losses (**Figure 7b**). In this chapter, we will evaluate whether it is feasible to enhance the olfactory doing through electric guidance of charged particles with charge levels and electric potentials that are safe to humans.

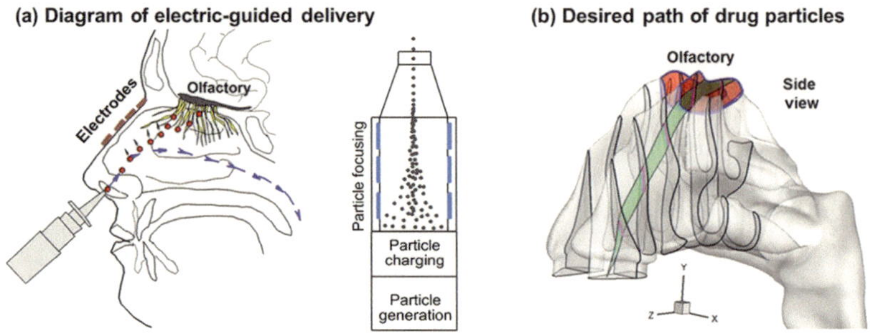

Figure 7. Diagram of electric-guided olfactory drug delivery. (a) Charged particles will be attracted toward the olfactory region by an applied electric field. (b) For optimal olfactory drug delivery, particles should travel along the middle plane of the nasal passage.

3.3.2. Idealized 2-D nose model

The proposed delivery protocol was first evaluated in an idealized 2-D nose configuration. The inhaled airflow field in the nose is shown in **Figure 8a**. There are three streams due to the obstruction of the inferior and middle turbinate. The upper flow stream is further divided by the superior turbinate. Only a small fraction of inhaled airflow was ventilated into the uppermost olfactory region. Due to poor olfactory ventilations, inhaled particles are unlikely to be conveyed to the olfactory region by convection or inertia. It is also observed in **Figure 8a** that stream traces initiating from the posterior naris move toward the nasal floor, while those from the anterior naris move toward the upper passage (superior meatus). It is hypothesized that pharmaceutical agents released into the at the naris tip have a larger chance to deposit into the olfactory mucosa.

To generate a desirable external electric field, four electrodes were put on top of the nose. The electrode voltages were specified to be −3, −8, −12, and 0 V, respectively (**Figure 8a**). The small electric potential (3 V) above the nasal vestibule was intended to impart particles an upward attraction. The electric potential above the middle nose was increased to −8 V to attract particles further toward the olfactory mucosa. The electric potential close to the olfactory region was around −12 V in order to catch the charged aerosols. **Figure 8b** shows the numerically predicted electric field (E-field), which changes from nearly 0 V at the nostrils to about −12 V at the olfactory region.

From **Figure 8c**, electric guidance of charged particles significantly increased the olfactory dosing, which was two orders of magnitude higher in comparison with that when an electric field was absent. **Figure 8d** displays particle transport in the nose 1 second after administration. The majority of particles (~95%) deposit in the olfactory mucosa. As a comparison, only 0.77% deposit in the olfactory region without an electric field.

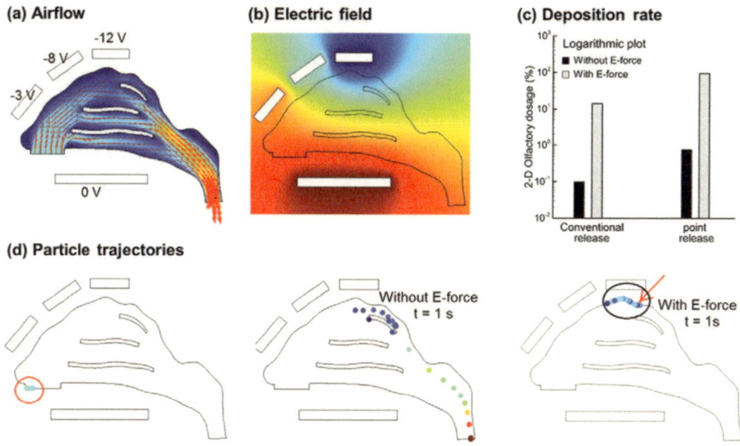

Figure 8. Computational modeling of electric-guided delivery in a 2-D nose model. (a) Airflow field, (b) electric field, (c) comparison of the olfactory deposition rates with and without electric guidance for conventional and point-release delivery techniques, and (d) particle trajectories with and without electric force for the point-release technique. Electric-guided delivery of charged particles can enhance the olfactory doses by two orders of magnitude relative to the case without an electric field.

3.3.3. *Realistic 3-D nose model*

A comparison of deposition patterns in the image-based 3-D nose model with and without electric guidance is shown in **Figure 9a**. The charge number of the particles is 5000, and the particle size is 0.5 μm. With an appropriate electric field, 3.7% of inhaled particles reached the olfactory mucosa (**Figure 9a**). However, only 0.06% of administered aerosols delivered to the olfactory mucosa without electric guidance.

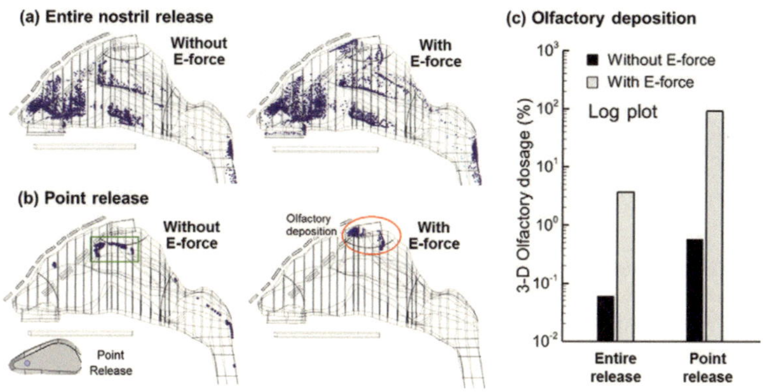

Figure 9. Computational modeling of electric-guided delivery in an anatomically accurate 3-D nose model. Particle deposition patterns were compared with and without electric forces for (a) the entire nostril release method (conventional delivery) and (b) the point-release method. (c) Significantly improved olfactory doses were achieved with electric guidance for both the conventional and point-release techniques. Electric-guided delivery increased the olfactory doses by approximately two orders of magnitude than without an electric field.

To further improve drug delivery to the olfactory mucosa, particles are released into a small point in the anterior nostril to minimize the filtration by the nasal valve and turbinate. With appropriate electric field strength, a majority (92%) of administered particles were dispensed to the olfactory region (red ellipse) that would have otherwise landed in the upper posterior nose in the absence of an electric field (**Figure 9b**, right vs. left). A careful study of the deposition distribution in the upper nose (green square, **Figure 9b**) shows that more aerosols are deposited on the turbinate wall (outer side) than on the septum (inner side). To minimize deposition in the turbinate, a lateral force is required to keep the aerosols from depositing onto the turbinate.

3.4. *In vitro* experiments of electric-guided olfactory delivery

3.4.1. Normal inhalation delivery

Particle deposition of charge particles was assessed in the realistic nose replicas. In order to generate a desirable electric field, two positive electrodes (25 and 100 V) were placed above the nose, and one electrode was placed below the nose as the ground. **Figure 10** compares deposition patterns of particles without and with electrostatic charges. For neutral particles, most inhaled particles deposited in the anterior nose while a small amount of particles reached the olfactory mucosa, which resembles the droplet deposition pattern visualized by Sar-Gel images (**Figure 5**). By contrast, significantly improved olfactory dosing was measured for charged particles under an external electric field (blue-dashed ellipse, **Figure 10b**). Meanwhile, filtration by the nasal vestibule and valve region was perceivably lower.

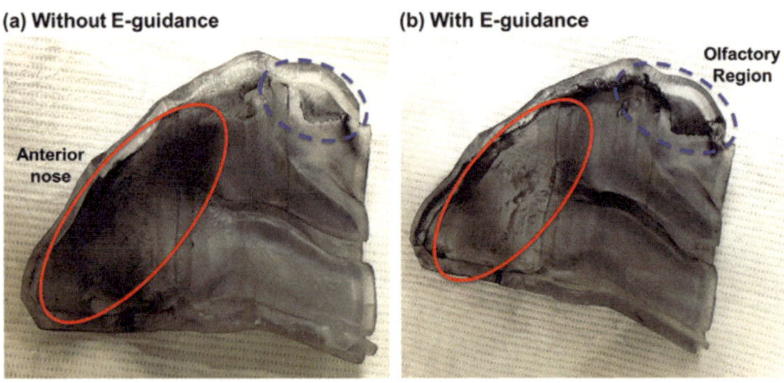

Figure 10. Particle deposition patterns in the 3-D nasal cast (a) without electric guidance versus (b) with electric guidance. Electric guidance of charged particles led to decreased deposition in the nasal valve region and noticeably enhanced deposition in the olfactory region.

3.4.2. Bi-directional delivery

The distribution of particle deposition using the bi-directional method is shown in **Figure 11**. High particle accumulations were observed in the upper nose of the right nasal passage, indicating there is an effective electric field guidance of charged particles to the olfactory region. It was also noted that particle deposition in the two passages was apparently different (right panel, **Figure 11**). In the right passage, particle deposition was more uniformly distributed, and a large portion of particles appeared to be pulled toward the electrodes. By contrast, the majority of particles in the left passage deposited in the inferior nose while much fewer particles reached the upper nose, presumably due to the gravitational effect.

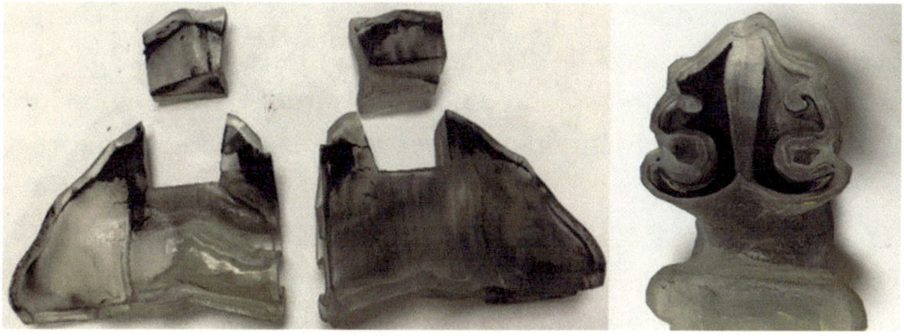

Figure 11. Deposition pattern in the right nasal passage and nasopharynx with the bi-directional delivery method. Appreciable deposition of particles was observed in the olfactory region. Because particles travel through the right and left passages in sequence, more particles were observed in the right passage than in the left passage.

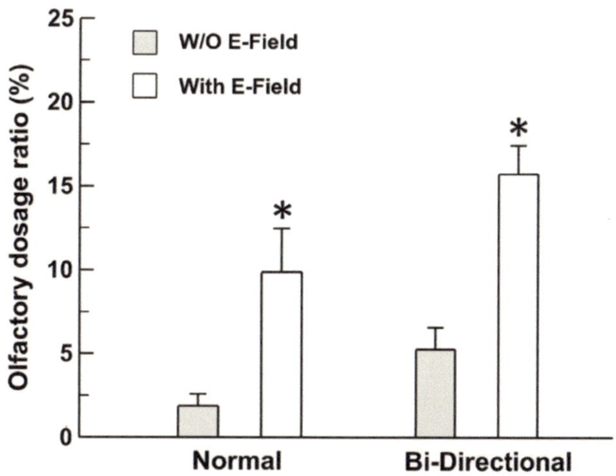

Figure 12. Comparison of the olfactory-to-nasal dosage ratio with and without electric guidance for the normal and bi-directional delivery strategies. *p-value < 0.05.

Figure 12 shows the comparison of the olfactory-to-nasal dosage ratio between the cases with and without the electric field guidance. The particle releasing time is 20 seconds, and the results are presented as the mean ± SD from five trials. With electric field guidance, significantly improved olfactory depositions were obtained for both delivery strategies, i.e., by a factor of 5 for the normal delivery and by a factor of 3 for the bi-directional delivery. The effect of the delivery method was also examined in the absence of an electric field; the olfactory dose using the bi-directional method was 2.8 times that under the normal method. However, with electric field guidance, the bi-directional olfactory dose was only 1.6 times the normal dose.

4. Discussion and conclusion

In this chapter, we presented a series of efforts in our lab aiming to improve the olfactory targeting of neurological medications. Both numerical and experimental tests were conducted to this aim by exploring various delivery strategies. Results of this study show that it is feasible to achieve clinically relevant olfactory doses using electric guidance of charged particles. All three protocols were demonstrated to give improved olfactory doses even though the improvement differs among the three. Compared to standard nasal devices, the point-release methods (vestibular and deep intubations) delivered approximately two order of magnitude higher doses to the olfactory region for both 150 nm and 1 μm particles. But even using the optimal delivery protocol (deep intubation), the olfactory dosage (1%) is still not adequate (~1%) to be clinically practical for the purpose of direct nose-to-brain drug delivery. In contrast, active control of drug particles using an externally applied electric field has been demonstrated to deliver much higher doses to target than the case without an electric field. An olfactory deposition fraction of 16% was measured with electric guidance under bi-directional breathing conditions.

The ability to dispense medications to the olfactory epithelium has tremendous superiority over convention inhalation devices in treating neurological diseases. A significantly enhanced olfactory dosing remits or eases the prevailing problem of too low olfactory doses. Second, reduced particle deposition in regions other than the olfactory region can minimize adverse side effects in those regions. Third, charged particles under the control of an external electric force will be are less dependent on respirations, making it suitable for seniors or subjects with comprised breathing capacities [52, 53]. The feature of robust delivery with electric guidance is especially appealing when the administration of medications requires long durations.

The electric delivery device is envisioned to have two major parts: a head-mounted nasal mask and a particle charging system. The nasal mask holds the electrodes and fixes the electrode relative to the patient head (**Figure 13a**). One example of the particle charging system is

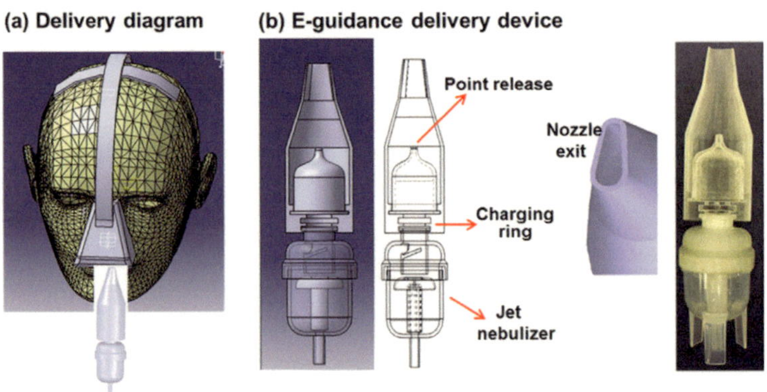

Figure 13. Electric-guidance olfactory delivery diagram and conceptual device designs. (a) A delivery system consists of two parts: a nose-mounted apparatus to generate desired electric field and a device to generate, charge, and point-release particles. (b) The conceptual delivery device uses a jet nebulizer and has an upright position.

illustrated in **Figure 13b** that contains a nebulizer, a charging ring, and a point-release nozzle. A prototype of this conceptual design was built using an Object30 Pro 3D printer (**Figure 13b**). An ideal design will generate small sized aerosols (<4 μm) at a slow speed and with high levels of electrostatic charges. Our preliminary test of this device, however, failed to produce such aerosols. Further testing and refinement are warranted to optimize the performance of this device.

Limitations of *in vitro* tests in this study include large particle size (30 μm), high exiting velocities of charge dry powders, large point-release area, and limited number of nasal models. Dry powders of 30 μm were selected because of the limited availability of dry powders satisfying both geometric and electrostatic requirements herein. Smaller aerosol particles are more sensitive to the guidance of electric forces and thus will lead to better doses in the olfactory region. A slow-moving particle will have longer residence time to respond to electric controls and is more likely to reach the target. In this study, the point-release catheter has a diameter of 4 mm and needs to be decreased to produce more site-specific doses. The nasal airway model was reconstructed from MRI images of one subject only and could not account intersubject variability. Future *in vitro* experiments and numerical simulations with more realistic scenarios are necessary to optimize the performance of electric-guidance delivery systems.

In conclusion, drug delivery of charged particles to the olfactory mucosa was assessed using both experiments and computations. Specific findings are as follows:

1. Complex nasal structure and no active control of particle motion in the nose are the two reasons lead to low doses in the olfactory region.

2. Conventional nasal devices, such as nasal drops, sprays, and nebulizers, fail to dispense clinically significant doses to the olfactory region.

3. The concomitant use of particle point release and electric field guidance can significantly enhance olfactory doses. With appropriate electric field and particle properties, a dose enhancement of two orders of magnitudes was predicted in both idealized 2-D and MRI-based 3-D nose models.

4. *In vitro* tests demonstrated a significantly higher olfactory dose using electric field guidance. There was a 5.2-fold increase for the normal delivery strategy and a 3.0-fold increase for the bi-directional strategy.

5. Future studies to refine the aerosol generation, charging, releasing, and guidance systems are warranted to further enhance the olfactory delivery.

Acknowledgements

Jun Lu at Central Michigan University, Linlin Zhao at Rutgers University, and Biwei Cao at Georgetown University are gratefully acknowledged for helpful discussions and for reviewing the manuscript.

Author details

Jinxiang Xi[1*] and Xiuhua April Si[2]

*Address all correspondence to: xi1j@cmich.edu

1 School of Engineering and Technology, Central Michigan University, Mount Pleasant, MI, USA

2 Department of Mechanical Engineering, California Baptist University, Riverside, CA, USA

References

[1] Bagger M, Bechgaard E. A microdialysis model to examine nasal drug delivery and olfactory absorption in rats using lidocaine hydrochloride as a model drug. Int. J. Pharm. 2004; 269: 311–322. doi: 10.1016/j.ijphann.2003.09.017

[2] Misra A, Kher G. Drug delivery systems from nose to brain. Curr. Pharm. Biotechnol. 2012; 13: 2355–2379. doi: 10.2174/138920112803341752

[3] Mistry A, Stolnik S, Illum L. Nanoparticles for direct nose-to-brain delivery of drugs. Int. J. Pharm. 2009; 379: 146–157. doi: 10.1016/j.ijpharm.2009.06.019

[4] Alam S, Khan ZI, Mustafa G, Kumar M, Islam F, Bhatnagar A, et al. Development and evaluation of thymoquinone-encapsulated chitosan nanoparticles for nose-to-brain targeting: a pharmacoscintigraphic study. Int. J. Nanomed. 2012; 7: 5705–5718. doi: 10.2147/ijn.s35329

[5] Shi H, Kleinstreuer C, Zhang Z. Laminar airflow and nanoparticle or vapor deposition in a human nasal cavity model. J. Biomech. Eng. 2006; 128: 697–706. doi: 10.1115/1.2244574

[6] Si X, Xi J, Kim J, Zhou Y, Zhong H. Modeling of release position and ventilation effects on olfactory aerosol drug delivery. Respir. Physiol. Neurobiol. 2013; 186: 22–32. doi: 10.1016/j.resp.2012.12.005

[7] Si X, Xi J, Kim J. Effect of laryngopharyngeal anatomy on expiratory airflow and submicrometer particle deposition in human extrathoracic airways. Open J. Fluid D. 2013; 3: 286–301. doi: 10.4236/ojfd.2013.34036

[8] Xi J, Longest PW. Numerical predictions of submicrometer aerosol deposition in the nasal cavity using a novel drift flux approach. Int. J. Heat Mass Transf. 2008; 51: 5562–5577. doi: 10.1016/j.ijheatmasstransfer.2008.04.037

[9] Illum L. Nasal drug delivery: new developments and strategies. Drug Discov. Today. 2002; 7: 1184–1189. doi: 10.1016/s1359-6446(02)02529-1

[10] El Taoum KK, Xi J, Kim JW, Berlinski A. In vitro evaluation of aerosols delivered via the nasal route. Respir. Care. 2015; 60: 1015–1025. doi: 10.4187/respcare.03606

[11] Wang J, Bentz J, Anderson R. Nasal device for delivery to the olfactory region. US 20070119451 A1. 2007.

[12] Gizurarson S. Method for administration of active substances to the olfactory region. Patents CA 2298596. 2003.

[13] Hoekman JD, Ho RJY. Effects of localized hydrophilic mannitol and hydrophobic nelfinavir administration targeted to olfactory epithelium on brain distribution. AAPS Pharmscitech. 2011; 12: 534–543. doi: 10.1208/s12249-011-9614-1

[14] Corley RA, Kabilan S, Kuprat AP, Carson JP, Minard KR, Jacob RE, et al. Comparative computational modeling of airflows and vapor dosimetry in the respiratory tracts of rat, monkey, and human. Toxicol. Sci. 2012; 128: 500–516. doi: 10.1093/toxsci/kfs168

[15] Xi J, Kim J, Si XA, Corley RA, Zhou Y. Modeling of inertial depositions in scaled models of rat and human nasal airways: towards in vitro regional dosimetry in small animals. J. Aerosol Sci. 2015; 99: 78–93. doi: 10.1016/j.jaerosci.2016.01.013

[16] Wilson IB. The deposition of charged particles in tubes, with reference to the retention of therapeutic aerosols in the human lung. J. Colloid Sci. 1947; 2: 271–276. doi: 10.1016/ 0095-8522(47)90028-7

[17] Bailey AG, Hashish AH, Williams TJ. Drug delivery by inhalation of charged particles. J. Electrostat. 1998; 44: 3–10. doi: 10.1016/S0304-3886(98)00017-5

[18] Wong J, Chan HK, Kwok PC. Electrostatics in pharmaceutical aerosols for inhalation. Ther. Deliv. 2013; 4: 981–1002. doi: 10.4155/tde.13.70

[19] Yu CP. Theories of electrostatic lung deposition of inhaled aerosols. Ann. Occup. Hyg. 1985; 29: 219–227. doi: 10.1093/annhyg/29.2.219

[20] Ferin J, Mercer TT, Leach LJ. The effect of aerosol charge on the deposition and clearance of TiO2 particles in rats. Environ. Res. 1983; 31: 148–151. doi: 10.1016/0013-9351 (83)90071-3

[21] Ali M, Reddy RN, Mazumder MK. Electrostatic charge effect on respirable aerosol particle deposition in a cadaver based throat cast replica. J. Electrostat. 2008; 66: 401–406. doi: 10.1016/j.elstat.2008.02.005

[22] Scheuch G, Gebhart J, Roth C. Uptake of electrical charges in the human respiratory tract during exposure to air loaded with negative ions. J. Aerosol Sci. 1990; 21: S439–S442. doi: 10.1016/0021-8502(90)90275-3

[23] Azhdarzadeh M, Olfert JS, Vehring R, Finlay WH. Effect of electrostatic charge on oral-extrathoracic deposition for uniformly charged monodisperse aerosols. J. Aerosol Sci. 2014; 68: 38–45. doi: 10.1016/j.jaerosci.2013.11.002

[24] Xi J, Si X, Longest W. Electrostatic charge effects on pharmaceutical aerosol deposition in human nasal-laryngeal airways. Pharmaceutics. 2014; 6: 26–35. doi: 10.3390/pharmaceutics6010026

[25] Xi J, Si XA, Gaide R. Electrophoretic particle guidance significantly enhances olfactory drug delivery: a easibility study. PLoS ONE. 2014; 9: e86593. doi: 10.1371/journal.pone.0086593

[26] Melandri C, Tarroni G, Prodi V, De Zaiacomo T, Formignani M, Lombardi CC. Deposition of charged particles in the human airways. J. Aerosol Sci. 1983; 14: 657–669. doi: 10.1016/0021-8502(83)90070-8

[27] Hashish AH, Bailey AG, Williams TJ. Selective deposition of pulsed charged aerosols in the human lung. J. Aerosol Med. 1994; 7: 167–171. doi: 10.1089/jam.1994.7.167

[28] Ali M. Engineered aerosol medicine and drug delivery methods for optimal respiratory therapy. Respir. Care. 2014; 59: 1608–1610. doi: 10.4187/respcare.03634

[29] Balachandran W, Machowski W, Gaura E, Hudson C. Control of drug aerosol in human airways using electrostatic forces. J. Electrostat. 1997; 40: 579–584. doi: 10.1016/S0304-3886(97)00106-X

[30] Djupesland PG, Skretting A, Winderen M, Holand T. Bi-directional nasal delivery of aerosols can prevent lung deposition. J. Aerosol Med. Pulm. Drug Deliv. 2004; 17: 249–259. doi: 10.1089/0894268042176355

[31] Luthringer R, Djupesland PG, Sheldrake CD, Flint A, Boeijinga P, Danjou P, et al. Rapid absorption of sumatriptan powder and effects on glyceryl trinitrate model of headache following intranasal delivery using a novel bi-directional device. J. Pharm. Pharmacol. 2009; 61: 1219–1228. doi: 10.1211/jpp/61.09.0012

[32] Djupesland PG, Docekal P, Czech Migraine Investigators G. Intranasal sumatriptan powder delivered by a novel breath-actuated bi-directional device for the acute treatment of migraine: a randomised, placebo-controlled study. Cephalalgia. 2010; 30: 933–942. doi: 10.1177/0333102409359314

[33] Si X, Xi J. Modeling and simulations of olfactory drug delivery with passive and active controls of nasally inhaled pharmaceutical aerosols. J. Vis. Exp. 2016. 111:e53902. doi: 10.3791/53902

[34] Xi J, Longest PW, Martonen TB. Effects of the laryngeal jet on nano- and microparticle transport and deposition in an approximate model of the upper tracheobronchial airways. J. Appl. Physilo. 2008; 104: 1761–1777. doi: 10.1152/japplphysiol.01233.2007

[35] Xi J, Longest PW. Effects of oral airway geometry characteristics on the diffusional deposition of inhaled nanoparticles. J. Biomech. Eng. Trans. ASME. 2008; 130: 011008. doi: 10.011008.1115/1.2838039

[36] Xi J, Longest PW. Transport and deposition of micro-aerosols in realistic and simplified models of the oral airway. Ann. Biomed. Eng. 2007; 35: 560–581. doi: 10.1007/s10439-006-9245-y

[37] Xi J, Longest PW. Evaluation of a drift flux model for simulating submicrometer aerosol dynamics in human upper tracheobronchial airways. Ann. Biomed. Eng. 2008; 36: 1714–1734. doi: 10.1007/s10439-008-9552-6

[38] Longest PW, Vinchurkar S. Validating CFD predictions of respiratory aerosol deposition: effects of upstream transition and turbulence. J. Biomech. 2007; 40: 305–316. doi: 10.1016/j.jbiomech.2006.01.006

[39] Wilcox DC. Turbulence Modeling for CFD. 3rd ed. California: DCW Industries, Inc. 2006.

[40] Hinds WC. Aerosol Technology: Properties, Behavior, and Measurement of Airborne Particles. New York: John Wiley and Sons. 1999.

[41] Morsi SA, Alexander AJ. An investigation of particle trajectories in two-phase flow systems. J. Fluid Mech. 1972; 55: 193–208. doi: 10.1017/S0022112072001806

[42] Xi J, Longest PW. Characterization of submicrometer aerosol deposition in extrathoracic airways during nasal exhalation. Aerosol Sci. Technol. 2009; 43: 808–827. doi: 10.1007/s10439-008-9552-6

[43] Matida EA, Finlay WH, Grgic LB. Improved numerical simulation of aerosol deposition in an idealized mouth-throat. J. Aerosol Sci. 2004; 35: 1–19. doi: 10.1016/S0021-8502(03)00381-1

[44] Ribeiro P, Si X Section 2: Electric and Magnetic Circuit. In: Beaty HW, Fink DG, editors. Standard Handbook for Electrical Engineering. 16 ed: McGraw Hill, New York. 2012. pp. 2.1-2.58.

[45] Longest PW, Xi J. Effectiveness of direct Lagrangian tracking models for simulating nanoparticle deposition in the upper airways. Aerosol Sci. Technol. 2007; 41: 380–397. doi: 10.1080/02786820701203223

[46] Cheng YS, Su YF, Yeh HC, Swift DL. Deposition of thoron progeny in human head airways. Aerosol Sci. Technol. 1993; 18: 359–375. doi: 10.1080/02786829308959610

[47] Cheng KH, Cheng YS, Yeh HC, Swift DL. Deposition of ultrafine aerosols in the head airways during natural breathing and during simulated breath-holding using replicate human upper airway casts. Aerosol Sci. Technol. 1995; 23: 465–474. doi: 10.1080/02786829508965329

[48] Laube BL. Devices for aerosol delivery to treat sinusitis. J. Aerosol Med. 2007; 20: S5–S18. doi: 10.1089/jam.2007.0569

[49] Geller DE. Comparing clinical features of the nebulizer, metered-dose inhaler, and dry powder inhaler. Respir. Care. 2005; 50: 1313–1322.

[50] Covert D, Wiedensohler A, Russell L. Particle charging and transmission efficiencies of aerosol charge neutralizers. Aerosol Sci. Technol. 1997; 27: 206–214. doi: 10.1080/02786829708965467

[51] Zeng Y, von Klitzing R. Scaling of layer spacing of charged particles under slit-pore confinement: an effect of concentration or of effective particle diameter? J. Phys. Condens. Matter. 2012; 24: 464125. doi: 10.1088/0953-8984/24/46/464125

[52] Dhand R. Aerosol therapy in patients receiving noninvasive positive pressure ventilation. J. Aerosol Med. Pulm. Drug Deliv. 2012; 25: 63–78. doi: 10.1089/jamp.2011.0929

[53] Willis LD, Berlinski A. Survey of aerosol delivery techniques to spontaneously breathing tracheostomized children. Respir. Care. 2012; 57: 1234–1241. doi: 10.4187/respcare.01518

Chapter 6

Enhancement of Percutaneous Absorption on Skin by Plasma Drug Delivery Method

Kazuo Shimizu and Jaroslav Krištof

Additional information is available at the end of the chapter

http://dx.doi.org/10.5772/65116

Abstract

Transdermal drug delivery (TDD) is a painless method of low-dose drug delivery. The advantages and disadvantages of transdermal drug delivery methods are named and basic methods such as using chemical enhancers, iontophoresis and electrophoresis are introduced. One of the promising methods make use of plasma which is generated in atmospheric pressure mostly in volume or on surface dielectric barrier discharge (DBD) or in plasma jet. As the plasma produces various particles according to the used gas, UV radiation and heat, their effects on skin and barrier function are described. Improvement of transdermal drug delivery of hydrophilic drug galantamine hydrobromide (GaHBr) using microplasma electrode is introduced.

Keywords: microplasma, plasma jet, plasma drug delivery, skin, stratum corneum

1. Introduction of atmospheric plasma for medical application

Medical applications of atmospheric plasma have been intensively studied [1]. These studies have reported numerous applications, such as for sterilization [2, 3], decomposition of harmful substances [4] and surface treatments [5–7]. In recent years, this area of research has been focused on the practical utilization of atmospheric plasma in the medical filed, such as for blood coagulation [8, 9], wound healing [10–12] and cancer treatment [13–15]. On the other hand, dermatology is one area of medicine where atmospheric plasma applications are currently used in practice [16], such as in a device to treat acne or wrinkles [17] and to treat stretch marks in combination with ultrasonic waves [18, 19]. As explained above, various research and development efforts have been conducted in the application of plasma medicine; however, we do not yet know whether plasma irradiation can be used to treat various symptoms. Though, the basic mechanisms of cell response [13–15] and the bacterial sterilization process [2, 3] have been studied intensively, effectiveness of plasma medicine in treating depression, which is a social problem in contemporary countries such as Japan, and Alzheimer's disease, which is an increasing problem in aging societies, has not still been investigated. The use of plasma medicine to treat various other diseases, such as cerebral infarction and high blood pressure, also requires additional investigation. Reactive oxygen species (ROSs) and reactive nitrogen species (RNSs) could play important roles in the beneficial effects of plasma medicine. Mechanisms underlying these effects could be quite complicated because of the physiological activation in the body by ROS signalling [20]. Fundamental research to elucidate the cellular response is currently under investigation. In contrast, reactive species generated in plasma or exposed liquid medium have demonstrated efficacy for treating various cancers, but not for the previously mentioned mental disorders, other associated symptoms or diseases such as diabetes, cerebral infarction and high blood pressure [21]. Fortunately, mechanisms of depression and Alzheimer's disease have been revealed in detail. The inhibited production of neurotransmitters (serotonin, noradrenalin and dopamine) causes depression, and Alzheimer's disease occurs because of the deposition of a peptide called amyloid-ß on the cerebral cortex. Research and development of effective drugs for treating mental disorders are proceeding [22]. These drugs are administrated orally; however, the effects of many of these drugs are delayed because of absorption in the small intestine. Moreover, as is the case with oral administration, absorption of drugs in additional locations is different for each person. Thus, administration by injection is used if a precise or high dose of drugs is needed [23, 24]. Administration of poorly absorbed drugs is also the same. However, frequent injections are not desirable in the view of a patient's quality of life (QOL). We can point out the following questions to guide the future of plasma medicine and develop it into a strong tool for the treatment of various symptoms:

1. Is plasma medicine an effective method for treating various symptoms?

2. If not, what combination of drugs in addition to plasma irradiation will be required?

3. Can plasma irradiation be an effective method for drug administration?

As mentioned in many of the references, recent studies of plasma medicine are mostly focused on direct or indirect actions of the active species. Hence, clinical cases, such as Alzheimer's disease, diabetes, cerebral infarction and high blood pressure, have not yet been investigated to determine whether reactive species and plasma medicine could be an effective treatment. Applying plasma medicine for treatment of various symptoms, we have been considering plasma irradiation as a method to deliver appropriate drugs [25]. One instance of this use is the enhancement of percutaneous absorption by atmospheric microplasma irradiation. Percutaneous absorption is a drug administration method in which drugs are absorbed into the skin or body. In this sense, this method is similar to an injection; however, there is no need for a needle in plasma irradiation. Administering drugs in ways that do not require needles could increase patient QOL and reduce the rate of infections. In addition, percutaneous absorption has several advantages, such as preventing metabolism of the drug [24] and stabilizing the concentration of drug in the blood [26]. However, it has disadvantages as well, such as the limitation of the molecular weight of the drug [27] and the need for moderate solubility of the drug in lipids [28]. The stratum corneum layer inhibits drug penetration because the skin acts as a barrier to guard our body from foreign substances.

2. Advantages and disadvantages of TDD

Transdermal drug delivery (TDD) is an alternative to oral and parenteral routes of administration. It can offer some advantages over other methods of drug delivery [29, 30]:

1. Reduction of dosing frequency, due to longer duration of delivery.
2. Lower dosing of drugs.
3. Circumvention of first-pass inactivation by liver that can metabolize drugs.
4. Reduction of gastrointestinal irritation.
5. Lower probability of over or under dosing.
6. No pain.
7. No risk of infection by a contaminated needle or via wounds caused by a needle.
8. Suitable for patients with problems of swallowing.

Disadvantages of TTDS:

1. Only some drugs are permeable through the skin.
2. Limited to drugs with a daily dose 10 mg and less.
3. Slow drug delivery.
4. Possible skin irritation.

3. Stratum corneum structure

Stratum corneum, an upper layer of the skin, is a lipid-rich matrix with embedded corneocyte cells, which are dead keratinocytes. Corneocytes are tied together by a protein called corneodesmosome (**Figure 1**). Renewal of stratum corneum occurs every 14 days [31]. This layer is the first barrier for transdermal drug delivery. Lipid-rich matrix is used for transdermal drug delivery (TDD)—intercellular pathway. The lipid-rich matrix is composed of hydrophilic domain—head of ceramides and lipophilic domain—tails (**Figure 1**). The lipids in stratum corneum include mostly ceramides (41%), cholesterol (27%), cholesteryl esters (10%) and fatty acids (9%) with a small fraction of cholesterol sulphate (2%) [32]. The presence of ceramides indicates that lipids will be structured [31].

The permeability of stratum corneum lipid membranes depends strongly on the ceramide composition of these membranes. Molecular dynamics simulations show that ceramides with shorter (four- to eight-carbon acyl chains) fatty acid chains increase skin permeability, whereas further shortening of the chain leads to increased resistance to penetration almost as good as that of ceramides from healthy skin (24 carbons long on average) [33]. In order to enhance skin permeability, mechanisms like alternation of lipids of stratum corneum and its fluidity or creation of the disordering effect between alkyl chains of lipids of stratum corneum have been proposed [34].

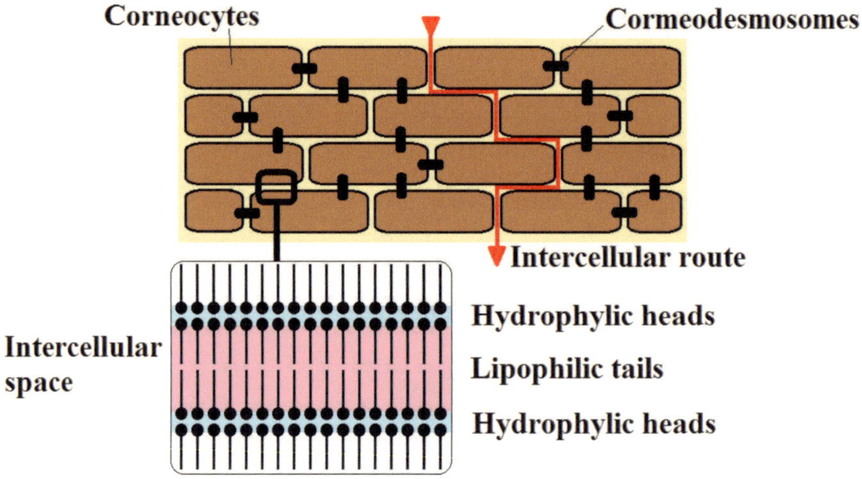

Figure 1. Stratum corneum layer with intercellular space [31].

4. Diagnostics of barrier properties of the skin—TEWL (transepidermal water loss), TST (tape stripping test), ATR-FTIR (attenuated total reflection-Fourier transform infrared spectroscopy)

There are wide varieties of methods available for analysing skin structure and other properties including its barrier function, such as Raman spectroscopy [35], X-ray diffraction [36], electron diffraction [37] and transmission electron microscopy [38]. Barrier properties of the stratum corneum can be confirmed by the transepidermal water loss (TEWL) test, which indicates water evaporation from the inner body through skin [21]. This test expresses the amount of water in grams evaporated per square metre in 1 h. Stratum corneum is a barrier against water diffusion and some other chemicals. The better the barrier function of the skin, the higher the water content and the lower the TEWL value. The tape striping test was described for the first time by Pinkus [39] in 1951. This method is based on removing of stratum corneum layers of the skin. The amount of removed stratum corneum is not constant and it depends on many parameters such as cohesion between cells, hydration or body sites [40]. This technique has been used for evaluation of the barrier function of skin, i.e. for investigating the depth of penetration of drugs [41], the influence of drug enhancers on stratum corneum [42], pH profiles [43] and many others. The tape stripping test (TST) is a representative method for estimating the barrier performance of skin and other properties of the stratum corneum [44]. When the

Scotch tape is placed on skin and peeled off, stratum corneum layer is stuck to the surface of the tape. Therefore, the barrier performance is decreased. Attenuated total reflection-Fourier transform infrared spectroscopy (ATR-FTIR) is an effective method when a material which is not well transmissive is measured, and the method can be used for liquid or solid samples. The information tells us about several micrometres of surface; thus, it is also a useful method for analysing skin [45, 46]. ATR-FTIR spectra can give us information about hydration of skin [47], structure of proteins [48] and lipids [49] and about their changes during skin treatment by chemical or other drug enhancers [50, 51]. There are several vibrational bands associated with chemical functional groups. Vibrational bands at 2850 and 2920 cm^{-1} belong to CH_2 symmetric and asymmetric stretching modes, respectively [52]. The absorbance of the spectrum decreases as the thickness of the skin decreases and the wavenumber indicates a change in chain conformation, especially a change in peak shape [49].

5. Introduction to chemical and physical transdermal drug delivery methods

The stratum corneum provides a barrier to any chemical entering the body and only small molecules having a molecular weight of less than 500 Da (Daltons) can passively diffuse through the skin at rates resulting in therapeutic effects. There are several methods for overcoming this barrier such as using chemical enhancers or physical ways using electric current or plasma discharge.

5.1. Chemical enhancers in transdermal drug delivery

Chemical enhancers are substances that change properties of skin for better penetration of drugs. The most well-known chemical enhancers are alcohols, fatty acids, terpenes and azone. An increase in permeability is very often caused by fluidising the lipids in stratum corneum. However, it is not valid for high concentration of short chain alcohols (like ethanol), where there was observed only a decrease of the absorbance of CH_2 stretching bands and no shift of their position; thus, there is only the extraction of lipids [53]. Many enhancers have long hydrocarbon chains, and it was found out that for fatty acids and fatty alcohols, enhancement is related to the length of the hydrophobic group chain [32]. Enhancer can interact with polar head or with hydrophobic tails of lipid bilayer or with proteins. Water increases fluidity of stratum corneum by insertion of water molecules between polar head groups. Dimethylsulfoxide (DMSO) interacts with intercellular lipids and keratin. Azone disrupts lipid structure, and oleic acid increases fluidity of intercellular lipids. The most effective enhancers are those which interact with lipids and also with proteins of stratum corneum [54]. Combinations of chemical enhancers have been used to maximize the effect of the permeability of drugs, and chemical enhancers are also combined with physical enhancing methods such as iontophoresis [55].

5.2. Iontophoresis in transdermal drug delivery

Iontophoresis (**Figure 2**) is a class of noninvasive methods to increase penetrations of ions through the skin by applying electric current using low voltages of up to 10 V (**Figure 2**).

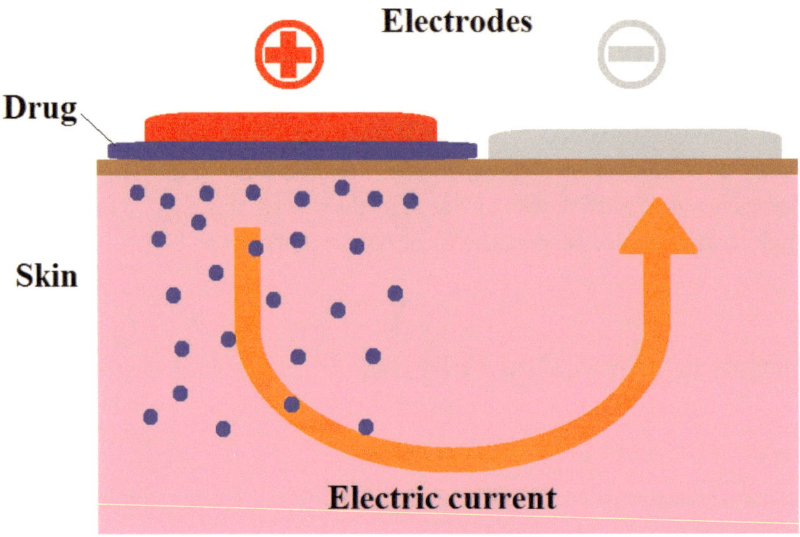

Figure 2. Application of iontophoresis to skin.

Various waveforms of applied current have been investigated [56], and it has been shown that various waveforms have various effectivities for skin permeability [57]. Iontophoresis enhances transdermal drug delivery by three mechanisms:

1. Ion-electric field interaction causing moving of drug (ions) away from the electrode through the skin.
2. Flow of electric current increases skin permeability.
3. Electro-osmosis caused by solvent flow from the anode to cathode because of negatively charged skin due to amino acids in cell membranes.

Iontophoresis is used for ionisable drugs, and it is most effective for molecules with weight of up to 7 kDa [58] or 10–15 kDa according to Kalluri and Banga [59]. The disadvantages of iontophoresis are: difficulties with stabilizing the therapeutic agent in the application vehicle, complexity of the drug release system and prolonged skin exposure to an electric current [60]. The main changes on skin after iontophoresis are an increase of the hydration of stratum corneum and a decrease of electrical resistance of the skin [61]. Analysis of asymmetric CH_2 peak, in ATR-FTIR spectra, did not show lipid alkyl chain disorders characterised by band shift or band broadening even at high current densities in some previous works [61–64]. On the other hand, in the recent work of Prasad et al. [65], they observed a shift of asymmetric CH_2 band with increasing of current density that achieved 8 cm^{-1} at 0.2 mA/cm^2. Also decreasing of lipid and protein bands intensity indicates lipid and protein extraction. The spectra also demonstrated a split in amide II band into 1553 and 1541 cm^{-1}. The split could be due to the disruption in hydrogen bonding associated with the head of ceramides, breaking interlamellar hydrogen bonding of the lipid bilayer and disrupting the barrier property of stratum corneum, resulting in loosening of lipid-protein domains, thus allowing higher flux as compared to the passive treatment [65]. Reversibility studies were conducted *in vivo* after 24 and 48 h of the application of iontophoresis. It was observed that the recovery process had started in 24 h and almost total recovery of epidermal as well as dermal changes was found in 48 h with low current density DC iontophoresis. However, with iontophoresis using 0.5 mA/cm^2 current density, edema along with focal disruption of the epidermis persisted [65].

5.3. Electroporation in transdermal drug delivery

Unlike iontophoresis, electroporation (**Figure 3**) uses high voltage (HV) (over 100 V) pulses for short time (in range of microseconds to milliseconds). Cells exposed to an electrical pulse open pores in the cell membrane and allow macromolecules to enter. It was confirmed that delivery of drugs of at least 40 kDa can be achieved [66]. The disadvantages of electroporation are as follows: (1) if the pulses have not adequate length and intensity, pores can be too large or cause cell damage, non-specific amount of material can be released to the cell [67]. (2) The created pores can persist for several hours, which allow a higher amount of drug to be delivered [30].

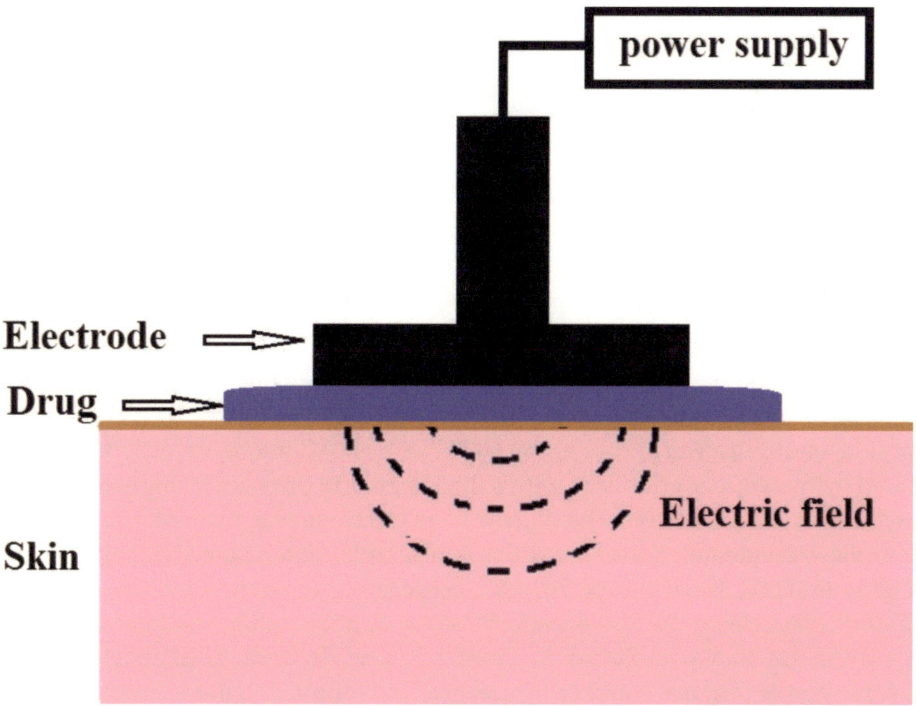

Figure 3. Application of electroporation application.

6. Plasma sources used for skin treatment

Several kinds of plasma sources were used for investigation of transdermal drug delivery so far, such as volume dielectric barrier discharge (DBD), surface DBD and plasma jet.

6.1. Volume DBD

Volume DBD (**Figure 4**) with one isolated electrode has been used in the study of Kalghatgi et al. [68]. Plasma can be with direct contact with a treated object (placed between electrodes) but with increasing distance of electrodes, ignition voltage also increases, too. This means that very high voltages need to be used in real applications. Kalghatgi et al. used pulsed discharge with a pulse duration of 1–10 μs. They applied 10 kV in the frequency range of 50–3.5 kHz to HV electrode isolated by quartz glass. The skin was treated from 15 to 120 s.

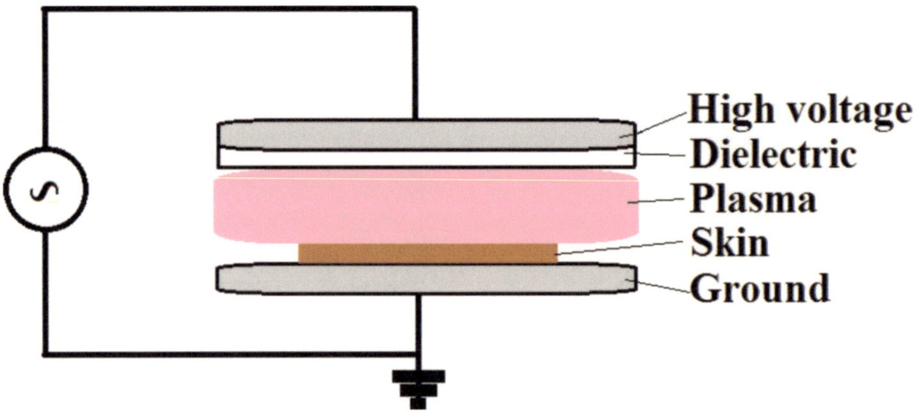

Figure 4. Volume dielectric barrier discharge.

6.2. Surface DBD

Another version of DBD is surface DBD used in Shimizu et al. [23, 69]. Both electrodes were in contact with isolator layer. Each electrode had a thickness in micrometre dimensions. These low dimensions allowed the decrease of ignition voltage to hundreds of volts. During treatment of skin, electrodes were powered by 600 V with an AC frequency of 27 kHz. Electrodes are created by two copper grids each with a thickness of 18 μm with insulation layer between them with thickness of 100 μm. The high-voltage electrode was covered with an insulation layer and the grounded electrode faced the skin samples at a distance of approximately 1.5 mm (**Figure 5**). Thus, there was no risk of electric shock to users, even when touching the surface of the film electrode. The waveform of the applied voltage and corresponding discharge current are shown in **Figure 5**. Holes between electrode lines allowed gas to pass towards the sample (**Figures 5** and **6**). Argon gas was supplied to the microplasma electrode systems with a flow rate of 5 L/min through the tube that was connected to the electrode. The exposure time was usually between 1 and 5 min (**Figure 7**).

http://dx.doi.org/10.5772/65116

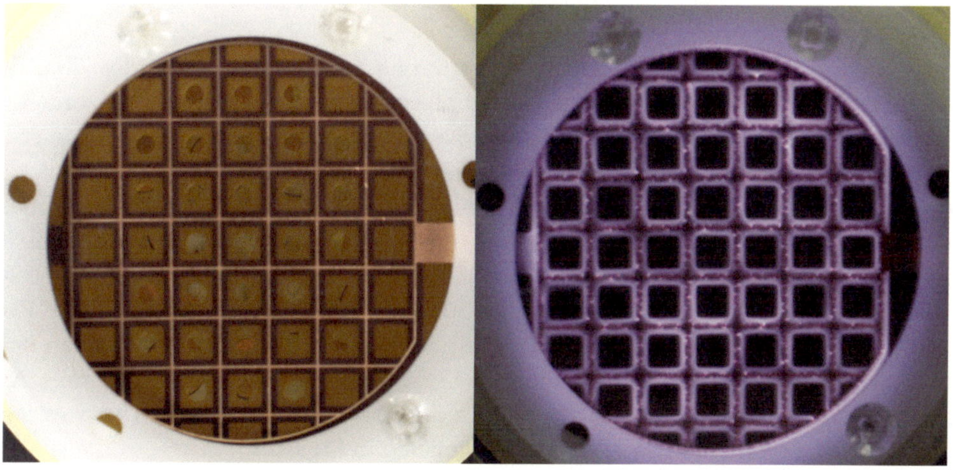

Figure 5. Top view of microplasma electrode, before discharge (left), discharge with Ar gas – 600 V (right) [69].

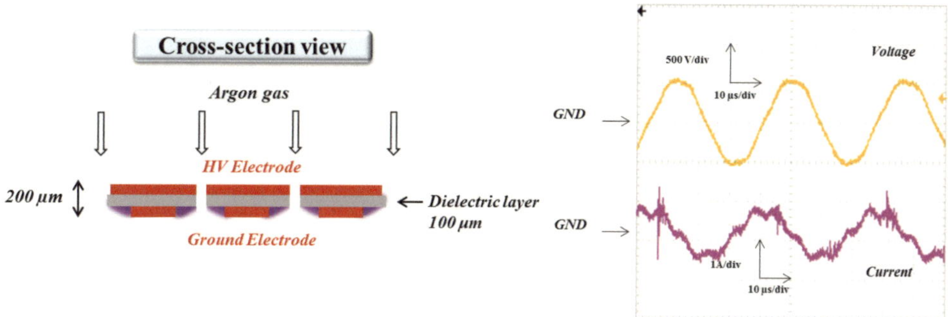

Figure 6. Cross section of microplasma electrode (left); waveforms of microplasma discharge (right) [69].

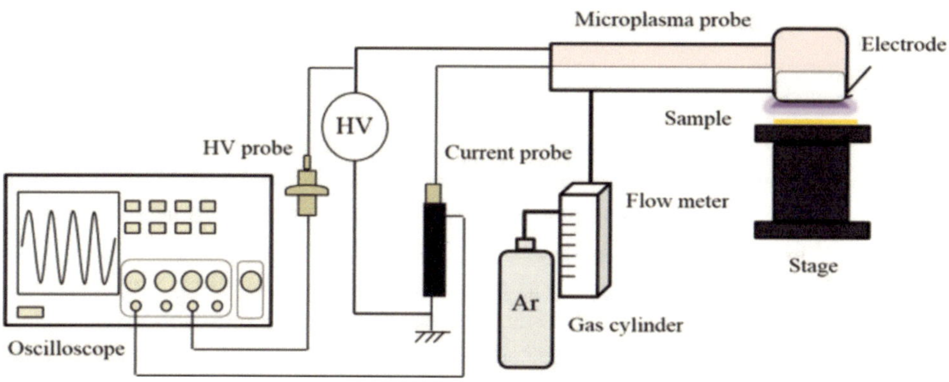

Figure 7. Experimental set-up with microplasma electrode [23].

6.3. Plasma jet

Plasma jets consist usually from a gas nozzle with one, two or three electrodes [70, 71]. The plasma jet can be realised by two ways—active plasma jets (expanding plasma contains free and high energetic electrons) and remote plasma jets (plasma is potential free and consists of relaxing and recombining active species from inside the nozzle) [70]. The plasma jet in **Figure 8** consists of a Pyrex tube and a central tungsten high voltage (HV) electrode. The grounded electrode is an aluminium ring located at the end of the outer surface of the Pyrex tube. The distance between the skin sample and the outlet of the plasma jet was set to 2 mm. The sample was isolated from the holder by a 30-mm thick PVC isolator or without isolator to compare the effect of the conductive layer under the skin surface as the human body is not isolator. The treatment time of the sample was set from several seconds to 1 min. Argon, nitrogen or argon-water vapour gases were introduced into the plasma jet. The waveform of the voltage and current of argon plasma jet is depicted in **Figure 8** [72].

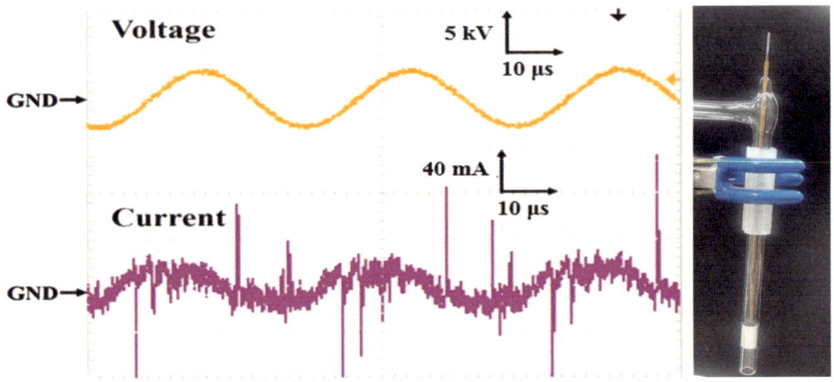

Figure 8. Waveform of plasma jet discharge (left) [72] and plasma jet electrode (right).

7. Plasma effects on skin barrier and transdermal drug delivery

7.1. Chemical reactions plasma particles with the skin

If argon plasma is used for skin treatment, the plasma produces electrons, argon ions, metastable and excited states. These particles can react with the skin directly. But, if argon or nitrogen plasma is working in atmospheric air, it makes the situation more complex because molecules of air (O_2, N_2, CO_2 and H_2O) can enter the volume of the plasma jet [73, 74]. In this case, argon can react with skin also indirectly through the excitation or dissociation or ionization process with air molecules. The reaction results in the creation of a number of species. It is difficult to find the molecule causing changes in skin. Pig skins treated by argon, nitrogen and argon/water plasma were compared by measuring ATR-FTIR spectra and monitoring of the shift of asymmetric stretching CH_2 band near 2920 cm^{-1}. A comparison of argon and nitrogen plasma jets has shown that argon can play a role in reactions with molecules of stratum corneum, but a similar effect can be achieved by nitrogen plasma itself as similar shift can be observed. A significantly higher value of shift was observed when argon with water vapours was used. The asymmetric stretching band was shifted 3.5 cm^{-1} (**Figure 9**). This result indicates that the stratum corneum became the most permeable after treatment of Ar plasma with water vapours. On the other hand, we observed low wavenumber shifts of the maxima of amide I and amide II (**Figure 9**).

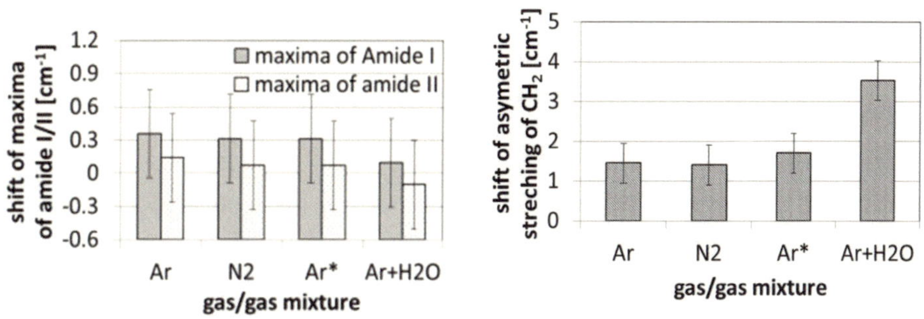

Figure 9. Shift of asymmetric stretching band of CH_2 to higher wavenumbers for the gases used in plasma jet discharge. Flow 10 L/min = (Ar*; N_2), 3 L/min = (Ar; Ar+H_2O).

Pig skin treated by argon microplasma shows shift of asymmetric stretching CH_2 band near 2920 cm^{-1} after 1, 3 and 5 min of irradiation comparable with the plasma jet (**Figure 10**).

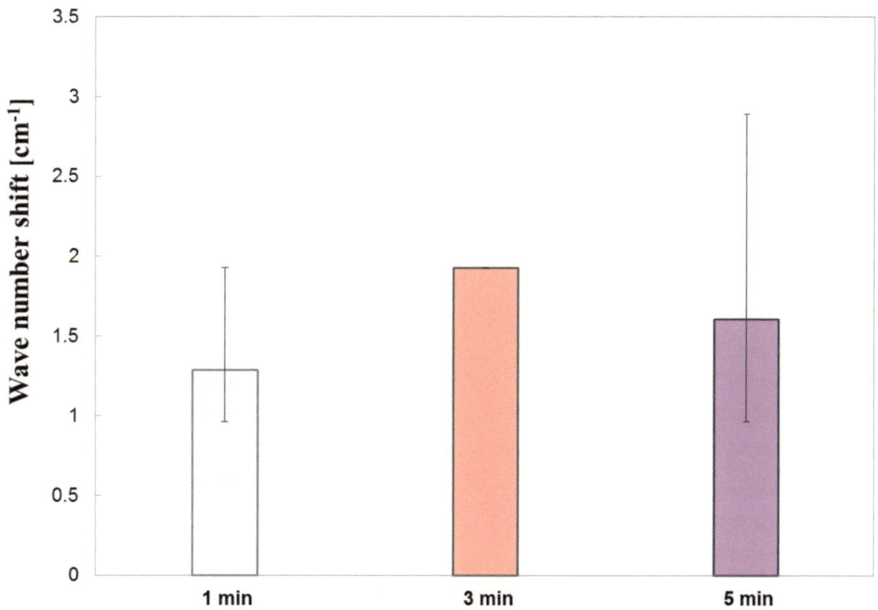

Figure 10. Shift of asymmetric stretching band of CH_2 to higher wavenumbers for Ar gas after microplasma irradiation [69].

When argon flew through the water reservoir, the argon ensured a higher concentration of water vapours in the discharge. The high shift of the asymmetric stretching band of CH_2 indicates that H_2O and the created OH molecules can play important roles in increasing the shift of the asymmetric stretching band of CH_2 in stratum corneum. OH could be created mainly by two channels [75]:

$$Ar_m + H_2O \rightarrow OH + H + Ar \tag{1}$$

$$H_2O + e \rightarrow OH + H + e \tag{2}$$

Simulation of the interaction of O and OH radicals with α-linolenic acid as a representative of fatty acid [76] showed that OH radicals most typically abstract an H atom from the fatty acids, which can lead to the creation of a double bond and also to the incorporation of alcohols or aldehyde groups, increasing hydrophilic properties of fatty acids and changing the lipid composition of the skin, causing an increase of skin permeability. Creation of these groups increases the hydrophilic character of the lipid layer. Incorporation of oxygen to stratum corneum lipids was also confirmed by increasing of C–O and C=O bonds after treatment of skin layer by atmospheric plasma [77]. Also, micropores (10 nm–1 μm in size) were observed in an artificial cell membrane system consisting of supported lipid bilayers after DBD plasma irradiation [78]. Later, it was found out that these micropores are induced transient species such as OH and OOH formed by plasma and they caused lipid peroxidation leading to truncated lipid chains, which induced pore formation [79]. These temporal pores were observed in skin after DBD plasma treatment and it was allowed to penetrate large molecules through the skin in several minutes. These pores had lifetimes of less than 5 min after treatment [68].

7.2. Effect of heating on skin barrier

Heating of the skin can increase permeability of stratum corneum [80]. Reasons of improving of transdermal delivery through the skin by increasing temperature are structural changes of stratum corneum lipids. Plasma can raise skin temperature from 30°C to more than 100°C which depends on the irradiated time, power of plasma source or used gas. Structural changes of stratum corneum lipids occur between 20 and 40°C, from orthorhombic to hexagonal ordered lipids. These changes can be indicated by CH_2 symmetric stretching frequency with an increase of 0.5 cm^{-1} in ATR-FTIR spectra or it is possible to observe by CH_2 scissoring mode where transition is revealed by splitting of the scissoring modes to produce a doublet with components at 1473 and 1463 cm^{-1}. Ordered lipid chains change to disordered chains at around 80–90°C. But some scientific groups identified more transitions in lipid structure [52]. For example, four phase transitions in temperature ranges 35–42°C, 65–75°C, 78–86°C and 90–115°C, respectively. Transitions below 75°C are reversible [81]. Between 35°C and 42°C two transitions can occur belonging to solid fluid transition and disruption of lipids covalently linked to corneocites at 37 and at 40°C to 'orthorhombic to hexagonal' change in structure. But too high a temperature can cause damage to the skin. Thermal conditions that cause burns of the skin are functions of the time and method of how the skin is exposed to the heat. Longer exposure of skin to a temperature higher than 43°C can lead to the formation of blisters [82]. It was found out that fast heating of skin can increase skin permeability without damaging deeper tissues. Investigation of high temperatures of up to 315°C applied to skin for 100 ms, 1 s and 5 s showed small variations between drug deliveries of calcein [82]. Exposure for 1 s or 5 s should be sufficient to equalize temperature in the full thickness of skin, but the 100 ms exposure should have influence only on stratum corneum. Between 100 and 150°C, permeability of skin was increased a few fold. This increase was attributed to lipid melting in the stratum corneum. In the range of 150–250°C, transdermal flux increased by two orders, attributable to disruption of stratum corneum keratin network structure. Above 300°C, transdermal flux increased by three orders, attributable to decomposition and vaporization of the stratum corneum [83].

7.3. Effect of UV radiation on skin barrier

The wavelength range of 100–400 nm is called UV light and is usually divided into three ranges: UVA (320–400 nm), UVB (280–320 nm) and UVC (100–280 nm). UV light can cause damage to skin. It is well-known that atmospheric plasma can generate wide range of UV light dependent on the used gas [84, 85]. UVC radiation can reach only stratum corneum and it consists of emission of excited NO molecule (200–280 nm—NO-gama system) or nitrogen molecule (120–200 nm—LBH system) in plasma discharges. The source of UVB radiation is emission of OH and nitrogen (second positive system of nitrogen). UVA is composed mostly of second positive system of nitrogen. UVA and UVB can reach deeper layers of skin like epidermis and UVA also dermis. UV radiation can cause formation of hydroxides and epoxides, hydrogenation of double bonds and breaking of carbon chains. The effect of UV on lipids depends on their structure, and only double bonds of fatty acids are sensitive to the formation of oxygenated molecules by oxygen in the air. These changes can be amplified or weakened by the surrounding atmosphere around the treated skin. When lipids of stratum corneum like cholesterol, cholesterol sulphate, ceramide III, linolenic acid and dipalmitoylphosphatidylcholine were irradiated by UV light up to 240 min, peroxidative changes occurred only in lipids with double bonds such as cholesterol and linolenic acid [86]. But the changes are not permanent and the order of stratum corneum lipids and water-loss protection can recover after 3 days and it returns to its initial state, thanks to repair processes in the skin [87]. Reactive oxygen species like superoxide anion radicals, singlet oxygen, hydrogen peroxide and hydroxyl radical can be created by UV light. For example, superoxide anion radicals are precursors to other oxygen reactive species, and it was found that there exists a correlation between the superoxide anion radical's concentration and degree of oxidation of lipids [88]. UV light is also used for treatment of some skin diseases but delivered doses have to be controlled and maintained in safety level to not penetrate to deeper layers of skin [89].

7.4. Acidifying effect of plasma on skin

Acidifying effect was observed after applying plasma to stripped lipids from stratum corneum. A higher decrease of pH was observed in discharges, which produced a higher amount of NO_x species. The same effect was observed on human skin, but after 30 min after plasma treatment, the pH of skin return to initial value [90]. The decrease of pH depends on parameters of the plasma discharge and the treatment time. Previous work has attributed the pH shift of water on plasma-treated lipids to the interaction of reactive species with the surface. Nitrates formed in water droplets could form nitric acid. NOx species could adhere on lipid surface or deposited nitric acid on the film surfaces by gaseous HNO_3 [91]. The recovery of pH in the post-plasma phase was attributed to the decrease of acidifying agents on the substrate surfaces by both diffusion and desorption processes.

7.5. Skin etching and skin damage by plasma

The etching effect of plasma is demonstrated in **Figure 11** by a cross section of the skin. The stratum corneum layer (the white part in (a) control sample) was removed after 20 tape stripping cycles, as shown in (b). After 30 s of atmospheric plasma jet irradiation, most of the stratum corneum layer was removed, as shown in (c). In the microplasma case, even after 5 min irradiation (d), the stratum corneum layer remained similar to the control sample, as shown in (a) [23]. Little difference in physical appearance was observed between the control pig skin sample and after microplasma irradiation. For the tape stripping test, surface asperity was decreased and after 10 s of atmospheric plasma jet irradiation, small pores (ranging from 40 to 100 μm) were observed. Physical damages on skin could be considered to arise from the electric field or an etching effect from bombardment with charged particles [92].

Surface potential can lead to a strong electric field across the skin and finally penetrate the skin to form holes. Holes were confirmed after longer operation (3–5 min) of atmospheric plasma irradiation. Pores and holes are shown in **Figure 12** after 10 and 30 s of operation of the plasma jet.

This physical damage could affect the barrier function of skin samples. When the effect of plasma jet was tested on PEN film, after 10 s of plasma jet irradiation, the surface potential increased to about 10% of the driven voltage. After long-term operation, it reached almost the same value as the driven voltage [23]. A similar problem could happen in electroporation but it uses very short operation times in the range of microseconds or milliseconds. High surface potential can induce current flow through the skin and it will increase the skin temperature and might affect cells of skin and cause thermal damage of skin [93]. On the contrary, the surface potential remained low in the microplasma case. The thickness of stratum corneum after 30 s of treatment of plasma jet is equivalent to 20 times of striping by tape. This is also confirmed by TEWL (**Figure 13**), which also shows the same values. On the other hand, TEWL after 5 min of microplasma irradiation of the pig skin sample, TEWL increased to almost double its original value, suggesting that the barrier properties were decreased through atmospheric microplasma irradiation but it is less effective than plasma jet [23].

http://dx.doi.org/10.5772/65116

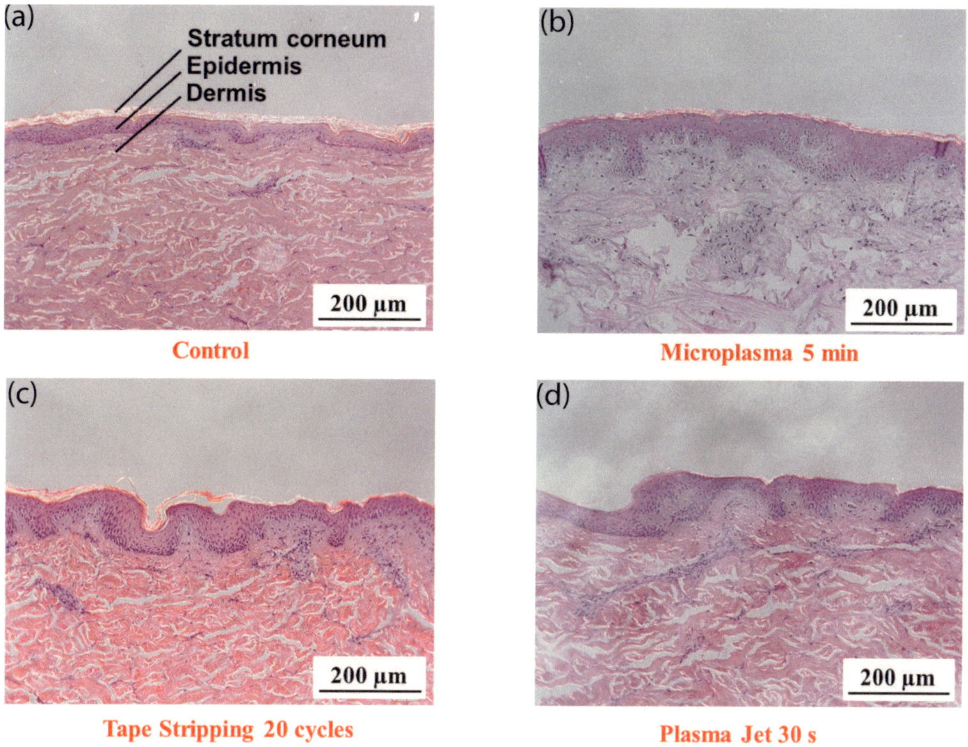

Figure 11. Cross section of pig skin after atmospheric plasma irradiation, and tape stripping test. (a) Control sample, stratum corneum thickness: 18.09 ± 1.64 μm; (b) tape stripping test — 20 times, stratum corneum thickness: 5.99 ± 1.24; (c) plasma jet — 30 s, stratum corneum thickness: 3.49 ± 0.61; (d) microplasma — 5 min, stratum corneum thickness: 13.40 ± 1.46 [72].

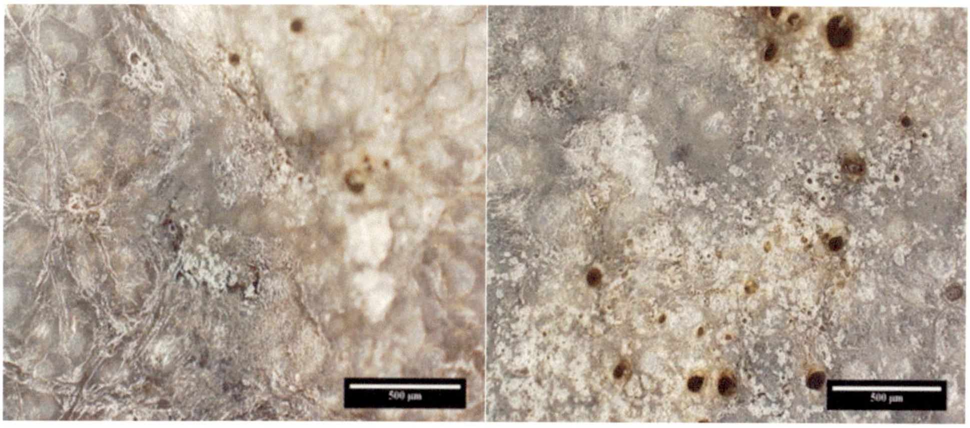

Figure 12. Left: 10 s of treatment by plasma jet; Right: 30 s of treatment by plasma jet [72].

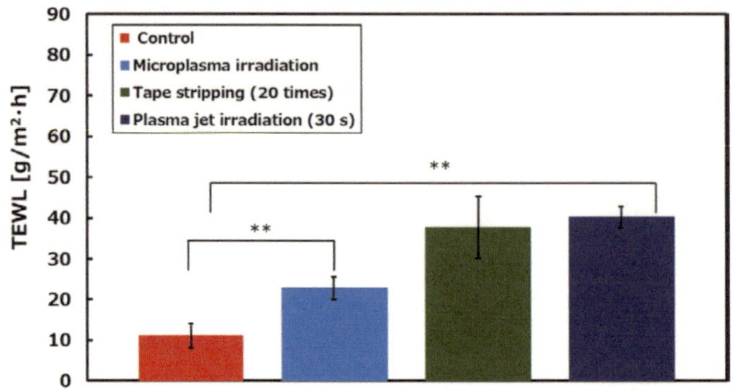

Figure 13. Variations of TEWL values before and after microplasma irradiation, tape striping test and plasma jet irradiation [72].

8. Improvement of galantamine hydrobromide (GaHBr) permeation by plasma irradiation

Galantamine hydrobromide (GaHBr) (**Figure 14**) is an alkaloid, isolated from plant species such as Narcissus and Lycoris species [93]. Treatment of Alzheimer's disease occurs by inhibition of acetylcholinesterase enzyme. The chemical structure of galantamine hydrobromide is shown in **Figure 14**.

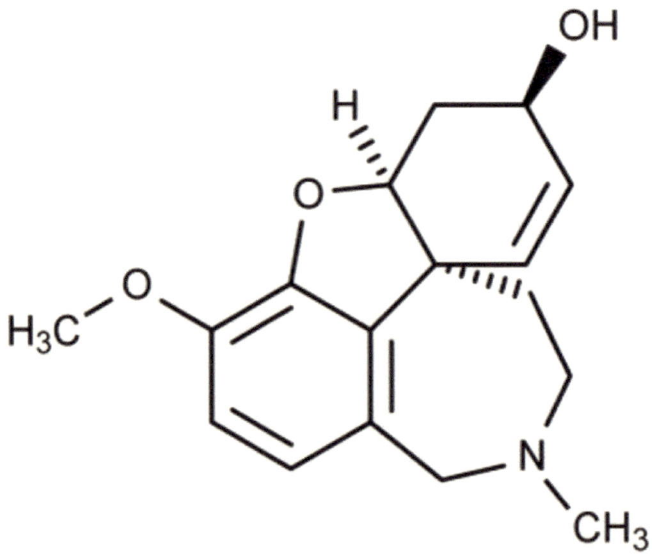

Figure 14. Chemical structure of galantamine hydrobromide.

As GaHBr is a hydrophilic molecule with a low molecular weight (368 Da), usually transdermal patches with chemical enhancers are used for transdermal delivery [94]. Using microplasma for the first time for enhancement of transdermal delivery of GaHBr, a slight improvement was observed with comparison of passive diffusion (**Figure 15**). Pig skin was irradiated for 3 min and then a water solution with GaHBr was applied on the skin. The permeation profiles of GaHBr through the pig skin delivered 5.35 ± 2.34 and 11.53 ± 2.89 μg/cm^2 for the control and the plasma-irradiated sample 24 h post-experiment, respectively [69]. These results lead to the expectation that microplasma discharge can be used to enhance the skin delivery of hydrophilic drugs and larger molecular drugs in the future.

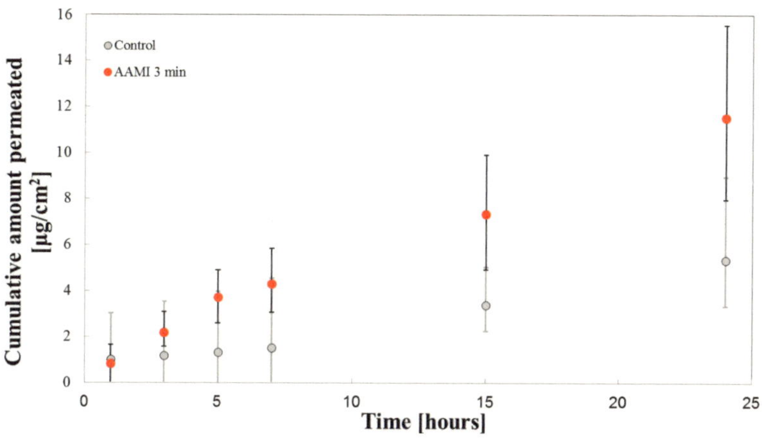

Figure 15. Amount of penetrated GaHBr—passive diffusion and after microplasma irradiation (red circles) [69].

9. Outlook of plasma drug delivery

Plasma as a source of UV light, heat, ions, reactive radicals and metastable states could be a successful tool for transdermal drug delivery. Each of these parameters can be used for improvement of skin permeability. Stratum corneum can be altered by chemical reaction of reactive oxygen species or by UV causing peroxidation of intercellular lipids. Undesirable heating effects can be tuned by the length of the plasma pulse and then a change of the conformation of lipids can be achieved also by increasing gas temperature in plasma. Improvement of permeability of skin by plasma was proved by ATR-FTIR and TEWL methods. A plasma jet is effective in etching of stratum corneum but can cause damage to skin because of the presence of a high electric field. We believe that plasma jet could be considered as a trade-off relationship, i.e. accompanied by physical damage or pain on the skin, similar to needles and creation of pores can cause risk of infection. On the other hand, microplasma seems to be more suitable for future drug delivery because it caused lower damage of skin. Transdermal drug delivery of galantamine hydrobromide by microplasma showed slight improvement in comparison with passive diffusion but further investigation is needed for drug testing or improvement in plasma properties in the future. We suggest that the use of a transdermal drug delivery with plasma irradiation is feasible, and thus, could be combined with appropriate drugs to target various symptoms such as Alzheimer's disease, diabetes and other symptoms that cannot be cured by applying plasma irradiation alone. This novel method will reveal new directions for the future of plasma medicine. Our aim is to combine a safe transdermal drug delivery method with a transdermal agent such as a peptide vaccine without requiring an injection needle and causing physical damage to the skin. Safety of patients, without causing harmful damage or physical damage to the skin, is critical for enabling this novel technology.

Acknowledgements

We would like to thank to Professor Akira Yamamoto and Dr. Kosuke Kusamori of Kyoto Pharmaceutical University, Professor Damon M. Chandler, Ms. An N. Tran and Dr. Marius G. Blajan of Shizuoka University, for fruitful discussion. This work was supported by JSPS KAKENHI Grant Number JP16H04085.

Author details

Kazuo Shimizu* and Jaroslav Krištof

*Address all correspondence to: shimizu@cjr.shizuoka.ac.jp

Shizuoka University, Hamamatsu, Japan

References

[1] Fridman G, Friedman G, Gutsol A, Shekhter A B, Vasilets V N and Fridman A. Applied plasma medicine. Plasma Process. Polym. 2008;5:503–533. DOI: 10.1002/ppap.200700154

[2] Shimizu K, Blajan M and Tatematsu S. Basic study of remote disinfection and sterilization effect by using atmospheric microplasma. IEEE Trans. Indust. Appl. 2012; 48:1182–1188. DOI: 10.1109/TIA.2012.2199953

[3] Kim J E, Lee D U and Min S C. Microbial decontamination of red pepper powder by cold plasma. Food Microbiol. 2014;38:128–136. DOI: 10.1016/j.fm.2013.08.019

[4] Shimizu K, Blajan M and Kuwabara T. Removal of indoor air contaminant by atmospheric microplasma. IEEE Trans. Ind. 2011;47:2351–2358. DOI: 10.1109/TIA.2011.2168509

[5] Pankaj S K, Ferrer C B, Misra N N, O'Neill L, Jimenez A, Bourke P and Cullen P J. Characterization of polylactic acid films for food packaging as affected by dielectric barrier discharge atmospheric plasma. Innov. Food Sci. Emerg. Technol. 2014;21:107–113. DOI: 10.1016/j.ifset.2013.10.007

[6] Kostov K G, Nishime T M C, Castro A H R, Toth A and Hein L R O. Obtaining, structural, magnetic and corrosive properties of Nd–Fe–B alloy thin films on glass. Appl. Surf. Sci. 2014;314:30–39. DOI: 10.1016/j.apsusc.2014.06.143

[7] Shimizu K, Fukunaga H, Tatematsu S and Blajan M. Atmospheric microplasma application for surface modification of biomaterials. Japan. J. Appl. Phys. 2012; 51:11PJ01. DOI: 10.1143/JJAP.51.11PJ01

[8] Ponsky T A, Gasior A C, Parry J, Sharp S W, Boulanger S, Parry R, Ostlie D J and Peter S D S. Need for subsequent fundoplication after gastrostomy based on patient characteristics. J. Surg. Res. 2013;179:1–4. DOI: 10.1016/j.jss.2012.03.064

[9] Haertel B, Woedtke T V, Weltmann K D and Lindequist U. Non-thermal atmospheric-pressure plasma possible application in wound healing. Biomol. Ther. 2014;22:477–490. DOI: 10.4062/biomolther.2014.105

[10] Ishaq M, Evans M M and Ostrikov K K. Effect of atmospheric gas plasmas on cancer cell signaling. Int. J. Cancer. 2014;134:1517–1528. DOI: 10.1002/ijc.28323

[11] Ahn H J, Kim K I, Hoan N N, Kim C H, Moon E, Choi K S, Yang S S and Lee J S. Targeting cancer cells with reactive oxygen and nitrogen species generated by atmospheric-pressure air plasma. PLoS One. 2014;9:e86173. DOI: 10.1371/journal.pone.0086173

[12] Ikawa S, Kitano K and Hamaguchi S. Effects of pH on bacterial inactivation in aqueous solutions due to low-temperature atmospheric pressure plasma application. Plasma Process. Polym. 2010;7:33–42. DOI: 10.1002/ppap.200900090

[13] Tresp H, Hammer M U, Weltamn K D and Reuter S. Differential viability of eight human blood mononuclear cell subpopulations after plasma treatment. Plasma Med. 2013;3:1–13. DOI: 10.1615/PlasmaMed.2014008450

[14] Haertel B, Backer C, Schulze C, Funke A, Wurster M, Woedtke T V and Lindequist U. Plasma-based stimulation of biotechnological processes in *Ganoderma lucidum* mycelia as example for a eukaryotic organism. Plasma Med. 2014;4:17–28. DOI: 10.1615/PlasmaMed.2014011874

[15] Gaens W V and Bogaerts A. Reaction pathways of biomedically active species in an Ar plasma jet. Plasma Sources Sci. Technol. 2014;23:035015. DOI: 10.1088/0963-0252/23/3/035015

[16] Liu D X, Iza F, Wang X H, Kong M G and Rong M Z. He+O_2+H_2O plasmas as a source of reactive oxygen species. Appl. Phys. Lett. 2011;98:221501. DOI: 10.1063/1.3592775

[17] Heinlin J, Morfill G, Landthaler M, Stolz W, Isbary G, Zimmermann J L, Shimizu T and Karrer S. Plasma medicine: possible applications in dermatology. J Dtsch Dermatol Ges. 2010;8:968–976. DOI: 10.1111/j.1610-0387.2010.07495.x

[18] Bos J D and Meinardi M. The 500 Dalton rule for the skin penetration of chemical compounds and drugs. Exp. Dermatol. 2000;9:165–169. DOI: 10.1034/j.1600-0625.2000.009003165.x

[19] Flynn G L and Yalkowsky S H. Correlation and prediction of mass transport across membranes I: influence of alkyl chain length on flux-determining properties of barrier and diffusant. J. Pharm. Sci. 1972;61:838–852. DOI: 10.1002/jps.2600610603

[20] Wiechers J W. The barrier function of the skin in relation to percutaneous absorption of drugs. Pharm. Weekblad. 1989;11:185–198. DOI: 10.1007/BF01959410

[21] Ya-Xian Z, Suetake T and Tagami H. Number of cell layers of the stratum corneum in normal skin - relationship to the anatomical location on the body, age, sex and physical parameters. Arch. Dermatol. Res. 1999;291:555–559. DOI: 10.1007/s004030050453

[22] Babaeva N Y and Kushner M J. Intracellular electric fields produced by dielectric barrier discharge treatment of skin. J. Phys. D: Appl. Phys. 2010;43:185206. DOI: 10.1088/0022-3727/43/18/185206

[23] Shimizu K, Hayashida K and Blajan M. Novel method to improve transdermal drug delivery by atmospheric microplasma irradiation. Biointerphases. 2015;10:029517. DOI: 10.1116/1.4919708

[24] Zorin S, Kuylenstierna F and Thulin H. In vitro test of nicotine's permeability through human skin. Risk evaluation and safety aspects. Am. Occup. Hyg. 1999;43:405–413. DOI: 10.1093/annhyg/43.6.405

[25] Suksaeree J, Charoenchai L, Madaka F, Monton C, Sakunpak A, Charoonratana T and Pichayakorn W. Zingiber cassumunar blended patches for skin application: formulation, physicochemical properties, and in vitro studies. Asian J. Pharm. Sci. 2015;10:341–349. DOI: 10.1016/j.ajps.2015.03.001

[26] Shen S, Liu S Z, Zhang Y S, Du M B, Liang A H, Song L H and Ye Z G. Compound antimalarial ethosomal cataplasm: preparation, evaluation, and mechanism of penetration enhancement. Int. J. Nanomed. 2015;10:4239–4253. DOI: 10.2147/IJN.S83402

[27] Franken A, Eloff F C, Du Plessis J and Du Plessis J L. In vitro permeation of metals through human skin: a review and recommendations. Chem. Res. Toxicol. 2015;28:2237–2249. DOI: 10.1021/acs.chemrestox.5b00421

[28] Klimundova J, Satinsky D, Sklenarova H and Solich P. Automation of simultaneous release tests of two substances by sequential injection chromatography coupled with Franz cell. Talanta. 2006;69:730–735. DOI: 10.1016/j.talanta.2005.11.011

[29] Jhawat V C, Saini V, Kamboj S and Maggon N. Transdermal drug delivery systems: approaches and advancements in drug absorption through skin. Int. J. Pharm. Sci. Rev. Res. 2013;20(1):47–56.

[30] Prausnitz M R and Langer R. Transdermal drug delivery. Nat Biotechnol. 2008;26:1261–1268. DOI: 10.1038/nbt.1504

[31] Hadgraft J and Lane M E. Skin: the ultimate interface. Phys. Chem. Chem. Phys. 2011;13:5215–5222. DOI: 10.1039/c0cp02943b

[32] Suhonen T M, Bouwstra J A and Urtti A. Chemical enhancement of percutaneous absorption in relation to stratum corneum structural alterations. J. Controlled Release. 1999;59:149–161. DOI: 10.1016/S0168-3659(98)00187-4

[33] Paloncyova M,Vavrova K, Sovova Z, DeVane R, Otyepka M and Berka K. Structural changes in ceramide bilayers rationalize increased permeation through stratum corneum models with shorter acyl tails. J. Phys. Chem. B. 2015;119:9811–9819. DOI: 10.1021/acs.jpcb.5b05522

[34] Moghadam S H, Saliaj E, Wettig S D, Dong Ch, Ivanova M V, Huzil J T and Foldvari M. Effect of chemical permeation enhancers on stratum corneum barrier lipid organizational structure and interferon alpha permeability. Mol. Pharmaceutics. 2013;10:2248–2260. DOI: 10.1021/mp300441c

[35] Caspers P J, Lucassen G W, Wolthuis R, Bruining H A and Puppels G J. In vitro and in vivo Raman spectroscopy of human skin. Biospectroscopy. 1998;4:S31–S39. DOI: 10.1002/(SICI)1520-6343(1998)4:5+<S31::AID-BSPY4>3.0.CO;2-M

[36] Bouwstra J A, Gooris G S, Weerheim A, Kempenaar J and Ponec M. Characterization of stratum corneum structure in reconstructed epidermis by X-ray diffraction. J. Lipid Res. 1995;36:496–504.

[37] Nakazawa H, Imai T, Hatta I, Sakai S, Inoue S and Kato S. Low-flux electron diffraction study for the intercellular lipid organization on a human corneocyte. BBA-Biomembranes. 2013;1828:1424–1431. DOI: 10.1016/j.bbamem.2013.02.001

[38] Honeywell-Nguyen P L, de Graaff A M, Groenink H W and Bouwstra J A. The in vivo and in vitro interactions of elastic and rigid vesicles with human skin. Biochim Biophys Acta. 2002;1573:140–130. DOI: 10.1016/s0304-4165(02)00415-4

[39] Pinkus H. Examination of the epidermis by the strip method of removing horny layers. I. Observations on thickness of the horny layer, and on mitotic activity after stripping. J Invest Dermatol. 1951;16:383–386. DOI: 10.1038/jid.1951.45

[40] Escobar-Chávez J J, Merino-Sanjuán V, López-Cervantes M, Urban-Morlan Z, Piñón-Segundo E, Quintanar-Guerrero D and Ganem-Quintanar A. The tape-stripping technique as a method for drug quantification in skin. J Pharm Pharm Sci. 2008;11:104–130.

[41] Pardeike J, Hommoss A and Müller R H. Lipid nanoparticles (SLN, NLC) in cosmetic and pharmaceutical dermal products. Int J Pharm. 2009;366:170–184. DOI: 10.1016/j.ijpharm.2008.10.003

[42] Bommannan D, Potts R and Guy R. Examination of stratum corneum barrier function in vivo by infrared spectroscopy. J. Invest. Dermatol. 1990;95:403–408. DOI: 10.1111/1523-1747.ep12555503

[43] Wagner H, Kostka K H, Lehr C M and Schaefer U F. pH profiles in human skin: influence of two in vitro test systems for drug delivery testing. Eur. J. Pharm. Biopharm. 2003;55:57–65. DOI: 10.1016/S0939-6411(02)00125-X

[44] Lawler J C, Davis M J and Griffith E C. Electrical characteristics of the skin. J. Invest. Dermatol. 1960;34:301–308. DOI: 10.1038/jid.1960.52

[45] Kazarian S G and Chan K. Applications of ATR-FTIR spectroscopic imaging to biomedical samples. BBA-Biomembranes. 2006;1758:858–867. DOI: 10.1016/j.bbamem.2006.02.011

[46] Chan K L A and Kazarian S G. Attenuated total reflection Fourier-transform infrared (ATR-FTIR) imaging of tissues and live cells. Chem. Soc. Rev. 2016;45:1850–1864. DOI: 10.1039/C5CS00515A

[47] Lucassen G W, van Veen G N A and Jansen A J. Band analysis of hydrated human skin stratum corneum attenuated total reflectance Fourier transform infrared spectra in vivo. J. Biomed. Opt. 1998;3:267–280. DOI: 10.1117/1.429890

[48] Karande P, Jain A, Ergun K, Kispersky V and Mitragotri S. Design principles of chemical penetration enhancers for transdermal drug delivery. Proc. Natl. Acad. Sci. U S A. 2005;102:4688–4693. DOI: 10.1073/pnas.0501176102

[49] Boncheva M, Damien F and Normand V. Molecular organization of the lipid matrix in intact Stratum corneum using ATR-FTIR spectroscopy. Biochim. Biophys. Acta. 2008;1778:1344–1355. DOI: 10.1016/j.bbamem.2008.01.022

[50] Zhang D, Wang H-J, Cui X-M and Wang C-X. Evaluations of imidazolium ionic liquids as novel skin permeation enhancers for drug transdermal delivery. Pharm. Dev. Technol. 2016;13:1–10. DOI: 10.3109/10837450.2015.1131718

[51] Balázs B, Sipos P, Danciu C, Avram S, Soica C, Dehelean C, Varju G, Erős G, Budai-Szűcs M, Berkó S and Csányi E. ATR-FTIR and Raman spectroscopic investigation of the electroporation-mediated transdermal delivery of a nanocarrier system containing an antitumour drug. Biomed. Optics Express. 2016;7:67–78. DOI: 10.1364/BOE.7.000067

[52] Mendelsohn R, Flach C R and Moore D J. Determination of molecular conformation and permeation in skin via IR spectroscopy, microscopy, and imaging. BBA-Biomembranes. 2006;1758:923–933. DOI: 10.1016/j.bbamem.2006.04.009

[53] Levang A K, Zhao K and Singh J. Effect of ethanol/propylene glycol on the in vitro percutaneous absorption of aspirin, biophysical changes and macroscopic barrier properties of the skin. Intl. J. Pharmaceut. 1999;181:255–263. DOI: 10.1016/S0378-5173(99)00055-1

[54] Barry B W. Penetration enhancers. Mode of action in human skin. J. Control. Release. 1987;6:85–97. DOI: 10.1016/0168-3659(87)90066-6

[55] Prasad R, Anand S, Khar R K, Dinda A K and Koul V. Studies on in vitro and in vivo transdermal flux enhancement of methotrexate by a combinational approach in comparison to oral delivery. Drug Dev. Ind. Pharm. 2009;35:1281–1292. DOI: 10.3109/03639040902882322

[56] Coston A F and Li J K-J. Iontophoresis: modeling, methodology, and evaluation. Cardiovasc. Eng. 2001;1:127–136. DOI: 10.1023/A:1014042109687

[57] Prasad R, Koul V, Anand S and Khar R K. Effect of DC/mDC iontophoresis and terpenes on transdermal permeation of methotrexate: In vitro study. Int. J. Pharm. 2007;333:70–78. DOI: 10.1016/j.ijpharm.2006.09.058

[58] Turner N G, Ferry L, Price M, Cullander C and Guy R H. Iontophoresis of poly-L-lysines: the role of molecular weight?. Pharm. Res. 1997;14:1322–1331 . DOI: 10.1023/A:1012100100865

[59] Kalluri H and Banga A K. Transdermal delivery of proteins. AAPS PharmSciTech. 2011;12:431–441. DOI: 10.1208/s12249-011-9601-6

[60] Krueger E, Junior J L C, Scheeren E M, Neves E B, Mulinari E and Nohama P. Iontophoresis: principles and applications. Fisioter Mov. 2014;27:469–481. DOI: 10.1590/0103-5150.027.003.AR02

[61] Jadoul A, Bouwstra J and Preat V. Effects of iontophoresis and electroporation on the stratum corneum: review of the biophysical studies. Adv. Drug Delivery Rev. 1999;35:89–105. DOI: 10.1016/S0169-409X(98)00065-9

[62] Thysman S, Van Neste D and Preat V. Noninvasive investigation of human skin after in vivo iontophoresis. Skin Pharmacol. 1995;8:229–236. DOI: 10.1159/000211352

[63] Jadoul A, Doucet J, Durand D and Preat V. Modifications induced on stratum corneum after in vitro iontophoresis: ATR-FTIR and X-ray scattering studies. J. Control. Release. 1996;42:165–173. DOI: 10.1016/0168-3659(96)01452-6

[64] Van der Geest R, Elshove D A R, Danhof M, Lavrijsen A P M and Bodde H E. Noninvasive assessment of skin barrier integrity and skin irritation following iontophoretic current application in humans. J. Control. Release. 1996;41:205–213. DOI: 10.1016/0168-3659(96)01329-6

[65] Prasad R, Anand S and Koul V. Biophysical assessment of DC iontophoresis and current density on transdermal permeation of methotrexate. Int. J. Pharm. Investig. 2011;1:234–237. DOI: 10.4103/2230-973X.93011

[66] Lombry C, Dujardin N and Preat V. Transdermal delivery of macromolecules using skin electroporation. Pharmaceut. Res. 2000;7:32–37. DOI: 10.1023/A:1007510323344

[67] Weaver J C and Chizmadzhev Y A. Theory of electroporation: a review. Biochem. Bioenerget. 1996;41:135–160. DOI: 10.1016/S0302-4598(96)05062-3

[68] Kalghatgi S, Tsai C, Gray R and Pappas D. Transdermal drug delivery using cold plasmas . In: 22nd Int'l Symposium on Plasma Chemistry; 5–10 July; Antwerp, Belgium. 2015. pp. O-22-6.

[69] Shimizu K, Tran A N, Kristof J and Blajan M G. Investigation of atmospheric microplasma for improving skin permeability. In: Proceedings of the 2016 Electrostatics Joint Conference; 13–18 June; Lafayette, USA. 2016. p. I4.

[70] Weltmann K D, Kindel E, von Woedtke T, Hähnel M, Stieber M and Brandenburg R. Atmospheric-pressure plasma sources: prospective tools for plasma medicine. Pure Appl. Chem. 2010;82:1223–1237. DOI: 10.1351/PAC-CON-09-10-35

[71] Stoffels E, Flikweert A J, Stoffels W W and Kroesen G M W. Plasma needle: a nondestructive atmospheric plasma source for fine surface treatment of (bio)materials. Plasma Sources Sci. Technol. 2002;11:383–388. DOI: 10.1088/0963-0252/11/4/304

[72] Shimizu K, Tran N A, Hayashida K and Blajan M. Comparison of atmospheric microplasma and plasma jet irradiation for increasing of skin permeability. J. Phys. D: Appl. Phys. 2016;49:315201. DOI: 10.1088/0022-3727/49/31/315201.

[73] Tsai I-H and Hsu C-C. Numerical simulation of downstream kinetics of an atmospheric pressure nitrogen plasma jet. IEEE Trans. Plasma Sci. 2010;38:3387–3392. DOI: 10.1007/s11090-013-9480-6

[74] Van Gaens W and Bogaerts A. Kinetic modelling for an atmospheric pressure argon plasma jet in humid air. J. Phys. D: Appl. Phys. 2013;46:275201. DOI: 10.1088/0022-3727/46/27/275201

[75] Bruggeman P and Schram D C. On OH production in water containing atmospheric pressure plasmas. Plasma Sources Sci. Technol. 2010;19:045025. DOI: 10.1088/0963-0252/19/4/045025

[76] Van der Paal J, Aernouts S, van Duin A C T, Neyts E C and Bogaerts A. Interaction of O and OH radicals with a simple model system for lipids in the skin barrier: a reactive molecular dynamics investigation for plasma medicine. J. Phys. D: Appl. Phys. 2013;46:395201. DOI: 10.1088/0022-3727/46/39/395201

[77] Marschewski M, Hirschberg J, Omairi T, Viol W, Emmert S and Maus-Friedrichs W. Electron spectroscopy analysis of the human skin barrier: cold atmospheric plasma-induces changes in lipid composition. Exp. Dermatol. 2012;21:921–925. DOI: 10.1111/exd.12043

[78] Tero R, Suda Y, Kato R, Tanoue H, and Takikawa H. Plasma irradiation of artificial cell membrane system at solid–liquid interface. Appl. Phys. Express. 2014;7:077001. DOI: 10.7567/APEX.7.077001

[79] Suda Y, Tero R, Yamashita R, Yusa K and Takikawa H. Reduction in lateral lipid mobility of lipid bilayer membrane by atmospheric pressure plasma irradiation. Jpn. J. Appl. Phys. 2016;55:03DF05. DOI: 10.7567/JJAP.55.03DF05

[80] Petersen K K, Rousing M L, Jensen C, Arendt-Nielsen L and Gazerani P. Effect of local controlled heat on transdermal delivery of nicotine. Int. J. Physiol. Pathophysiol. Pharmacol. 2011;3:236–242

[81] Wood D G, Brown M B and Jones S A. Understanding heat facilitated drug transport across human epidermis. Eur. J. Pharmaceut. Biopharmaceut. 2012;81:642–664. DOI: 10.1016/j.ejpb.2012.03.019

[82] Hao J, Ghosh P, Li S K, Newman B, Kasting G B and Raney S G. Heat effects on drug delivery across human skin. Expert Opin. Drug Delivery. 2016;13:755–768. DOI: 10.1517/17425247.2016.1136286

[83] Park J-H, Lee J-W, Kim Y-C and Prausnitz M R. The effect of heat on skin permeability. Int. J. Pharm. 2008;359:94–103. DOI: 10.1016/j.ijpharm.2008.03.032

[84] Yu L, Laux Ch O, Packan D M and Kruger C H. Direct-current glow discharges in atmospheric pressure air plasmas. J. Appl. Phys. 2002;91:2678–2689. DOI: 10.1063/1.1435421

[85] Sewraj N, Merbahi N, Gardou J P, Rodriguez Akerreta P and Marchal F. Electric and spectroscopic analysis of a pure nitrogen mono-filamentary dielectric barrier discharge (MF-DBD) at 760 Torr. J. Phys. D: Appl. Phys. 2011;44:145201. DOI: 10.1088/0022-3727/44/14/145201

[86] Trommer H, Plätzer M, Wolf R and Neubert R H H. Mass spectrometric examinations of stratum corneum lipid models exposed to ultraviolet irradiation. Skin Pharmacol. Appl. Skin. Physiol. 2003;16:291–304. DOI: 10.1159/000072069

[87] Merle C, Laugel C and Baillet-Guffroy A. Effect of UVA or UVB irradiation on cutaneous lipids in films or in solution. Photochem. Photobiol. 2010;86:553–562. DOI: 10.1111/j.1751-1097.2009.00690.x

[88] Kaneko T, Kaise Ch, Kimoto Y, Suzuki S, Kondo T and Yuasa M. Detection of superoxide anion radical in a stratum corneum intercellular lipid model using an electrochemical sensor. J. Oleo. Sci. 2011;60:647–654. DOI: 10.5650/jos.60.647

[89] Lademann J, Richter H, Alborova H, Humme D, Patzelt A, Kramer A, Weltmann K D, Hartmann B, Ottomann Ch, Fluhr J W, Hinz P, Hübner G and Lademann O. Risk assessment of the application of a plasma jet in dermatology. J. Biomed. Opt. 2009;14:054025. DOI: 10.1117/1.3247156

[90] Hirschberg J, Gerhard C, Braun A, Grottker S, Krupp A, Emmert S and Viöl W. Validation of the suitability of stripped lipid as a skin model in plasma medical investigations. Open J. Appl. Sci. 2015;5:40–49. DOI: 10.4236/ojapps.2015.52005

[91] Helmke A, Hoffmeister D, Mertens N, Emmert S, Schuette J and Vioel W. The acidification of lipid film surfaces by non-thermal DBD at atmospheric pressure in air. New J. Phys. 2009;11:115025. DOI: 10.1088/1367-2630/11/11/115025

[92] Babaeva N Y, Ning N, Graves D B and Kushner M J. Ion activation energy delivered to wounds by atmospheric pressure dielectric-barrier discharges: sputtering of lipid-like surfaces. J. Phys. D: Appl. Phys. 2012;45:115203. DOI: 10.1088/0022-3727/45/11/115203

[93] Martin G T, Pliquett U F and Weaver J C. Theoretical analysis of localized heating in human skin subjected to high voltage pulses. Bioelectrochemistry. 2002;57:55–64. DOI: 10.1016/S1567-5394(01)00176-1

[94] Yen W F, Basri M, Ahmad M and Ismail M. Formulation and evaluation of galantamine gel as drug reservoir in transdermal patch delivery system. Sci. World J. 2015;2015: 495271. DOI: 10.1155/2015/495271

Chapter 7

Biopolymer in Gene Delivery

Sakthivel Lakshmana Prabu and
Kandasamy Ruckmani

Additional information is available at the end of the chapter

http://dx.doi.org/10.5772/65694

Abstract

Nowadays, biopolymers, a class of biomaterials, represent frontier area in the drug delivery systems. Drug release from nano- and microparticles is a complex process, which involves several steps. Uptake of nanoparticle in the intracellular is affected by numerous factors. Recently, gene delivery has been considered one of the promising approaches for the treatment of various diseases acquired genetically in human being. The use of biopolymers as nanoparticles in gene delivery can potentially avoid many of the safety concerns in the gene delivery system. In gene delivery, the genetic materials such as DNA plasmids, RNA and siRNA are either encapsulated inside or conjugated to the nanoparticles, which protects the genetic materials until the drug reaches its target site. Treatment of the diseases is based on the effective delivery of the genetic materials into specific cells that are responsible for disease development. Various properties such as particle size, surface charge, morphology of the surface and release rate of the loaded molecules are the important parameters in the gene delivery system. In this chapter, various biopolymers (cationic polymers) and inorganic non-viral-delivery vectors used in gene delivery used as therapeutic agents are discussed.

Keywords: gene delivery, polymers, biopolymers, delivery system, therapeutic effect

1. Introduction

Polymers are the materials that are either prepared/produced synthetically or isolated from natural sources. Polymers can respond based on their environmental conditions such as pH, temperature, ionic strength, electric field, magnetic field, chemical and biological stimuli to deliver the desired therapeutic agents. Recently, biopolymer is a biomaterial used in various delivery systems to interact with the biological system and release the therapeutic agent. These biopolymers are utilized in the various applications due to their biocompatibility, biodegradability and low immunogenicity. Among the various biopolymers, synthetic polymers have well-defined structure and fine-tunable degradation kinetic and mechanical properties compared to the natural polymers. Recently, biodegradable nanoparticles have a major role in the field of health sciences especially for treating various diseases through drugs, vaccines and genes [1–7]. Nanoparticle in gene-delivery system has been utilized for treating various diseases such as cancer and haemophilia. The major challenge in the gene delivery is delivering the genetic materials such as DNA, plasmids, RNA and siRNA into the target/special cells to replace the damaged genes or expression inhibition of undesired genes or expression and production of required proteins. In gene delivery, the genetic material is either encapsulated inside the nanoparticle or conjugated to the nanoparticle. The nature, source and their physico-chemical properties of the polymers play an important role in the formation of desired properties of nanoparticles and to achieve a better therapeutic effect [8–12].

2. Polymeric gene delivery vector

The important property in polymeric vector is that the polymer should be non-toxic (biocompatible), biodegradable (hence have less toxicity) and also help to release the DNA from the complex into the cytoplasm. In polymeric vector, the polymer must be condensate with the genetic material. Condensate between the cationic polymer and genetic materials can be done through electrostatic interactions. By modifying the surface of NP, NP-DNA complexes can be formed by electrostatic binding between the positive charges of the NPs and the negative charges of the DNA. Only when the medium is aqueous and hydrophilic, the polymeric vector will be mobile, because the vector needs hydrophobic and hydrophilic components and be stabilized in an aqueous solution by forming micelles [13].

2.1. Polymer properties in polymeric gene delivery

Polymers have permanent cationic charges on its surface and are not preferred due to its strong condensate property with DNA, which will not release DNA into the cell. Hence, ionizable cationic polymers with pK values between 5 and 7 are preferred in the polymeric vector delivery which is shown in **Figure 1**.

Other important factors to be considered for the polymer in the polymeric gene-delivery vector are its molecular weight, molecular structure and composition of the polymer. Increase in the polymer's molecular weight also increases its toxicity. Polymers of different molecular structures such as linear, branched, stars and dendrimers have an impact on the transfer genes into cells [14–18].

2.2. Preparation of polymeric gene vector

Polymeric vectors are prepared by mixing plasmid DNA with a cationic polymer. During condensation between plasmid DNA and polycation, plasmid DNA undergoes a conformational change from a hydrodynamic size of 200–300 nm to particles of less than 100 nm. Plasmid DNA has a highly organized chemical structure [19–22]. A condensation between plasmid DNA and polycation is shown in **Figure 2**.

http://dx.doi.org/10.5772/65694

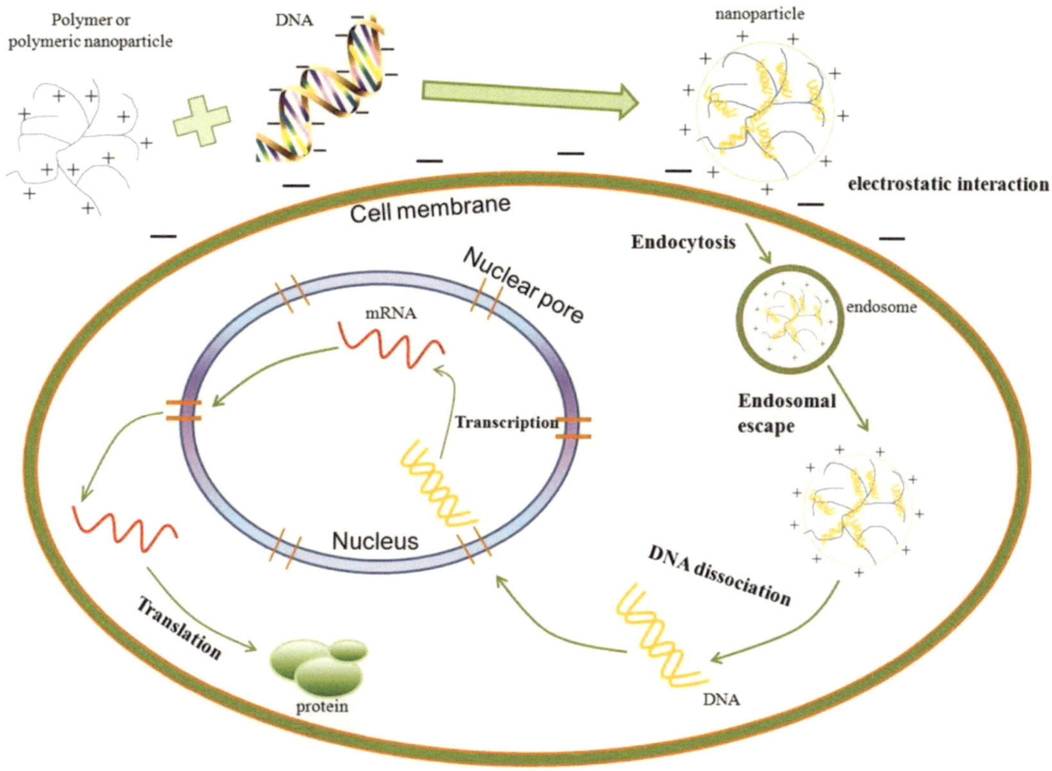

Figure 1. Gene delivery process of polymeric nanoparticle.

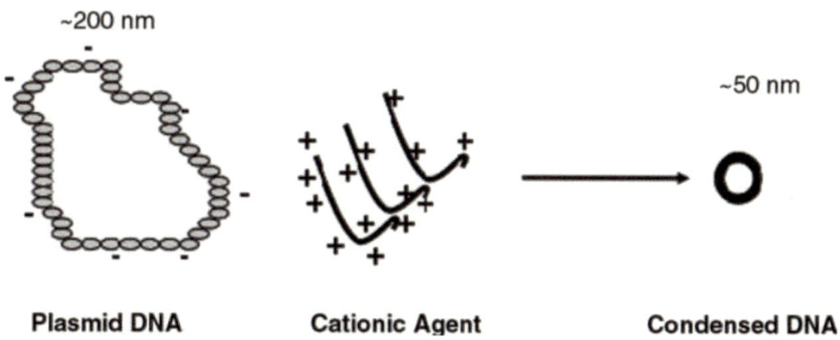

Figure 2. Condensation between plasmid DNA and polycation.

The order of mixing and vortex speed of mixing plays an important role in the size of the DNA nanoparticles. DNA can be condensate, either by evaporation under vacuum or by freeze drying. The freeze/thaw cycle can influence the particle size of DNA nanoparticles.

The charge ratio of DNA nanoparticles is the calculated ratio of amines on the polymer relative to the phosphates on DNA at a given stoichiometry of polymer to DNA. When a cationic polymer binds to plasmid DNA, sodium ions are displaced and the electronegative charge is partially satisfied. DNA condensates are normally prepared at near-neutral pH in low ionic strength buffer [23, 24].

3. Dendrimers

Dendrimer is a monodisperse macromolecule with perfectly branched regular structure and having at least one branched junction at each repeat unit 3. These dendrimers are used in gene delivery. The dendrimer/DNA complexes are encapsulated in a water-soluble polymer, and then deposited on or sandwiched in functional polymer films with a fast degradation by dehydration to mediate gene transfection.

Biodegradable dendrimers are commonly prepared by inclusion of ester groups in the polymer backbone, which will be chemically hydrolysed and/or enzymatically cleaved by esterases in physiological solutions. These dendrimers are large molecular weights which accumulate and retain in higher amounts in the tumour tissues. Dendrimer fragments are eliminated safely through urine.

Dendrimers are prepared through either a divergent method or a convergent method.

In the **divergent methods**, as given in **Figure 3**, dendrimer grows from a multifunctional core molecule to outwards. The first-generation dendrimers are derived from the core molecule that reacts with monomer molecules containing one reactive and two dormant groups. This periphery molecule is then activated to react with more monomers. This step is subsequently repetitive to produce layer-by-layer dendrimers for several generations.

In the` convergent approach, stepwise dendrimer is constructed, starting from the end groups and progressing inwards. The growing branched polymeric arms are called dendrons, which can attach to a multifunctional core molecule (**Figure 4**).

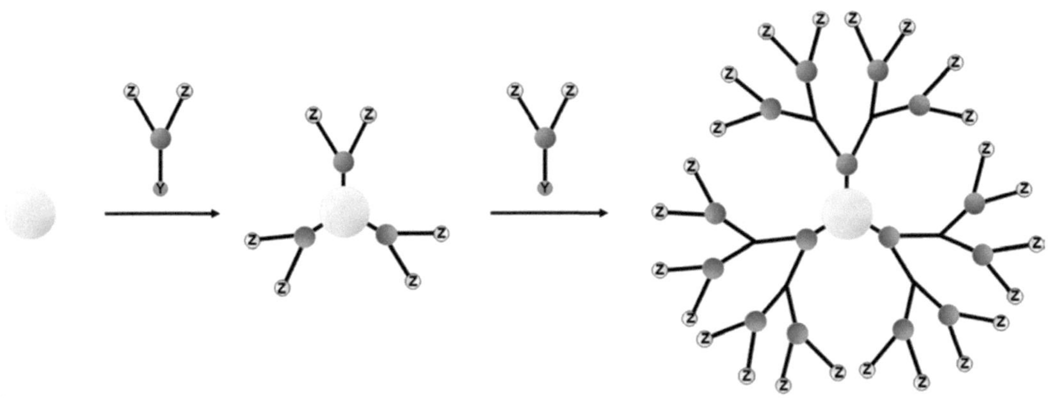

Figure 3. Formation of dendrimer by divergent methods.

http://dx.doi.org/10.5772/65694

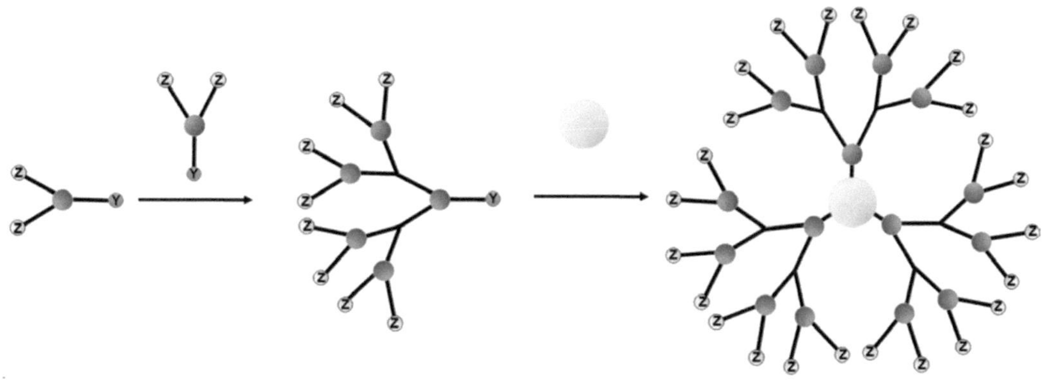

Figure 4. Formation of dendrimer by convergent method.

Whereas the structure Y in dendrimer is chemically active focal point and Z is the functional chemical group of another monomer.

3.1. Other types of dendrimers

3.1.1. Amino acid-based dendrimers

Amino acid-based dendrimers were developed to capitalize on the unique properties of the amino acid-building blocks, including chirality, hydrophilicity/hydrophobicity, biorecognition and optical properties. Optically active protein-mimetic dendrimers have been synthesized using various amino acids, such as tryptophan, phenylalanine, glutamic acid, aspartic acid, leucine, valine, glycine and alanine.

Amino acid-based dendrimers can be synthesized by

1. amino acid or peptide grafting and display on the surface of a conventional dendrimer
2. attachment of amino acids or peptides to an organic or a peptide core.

3.1.2. Glycodendrimers

Carbohydrate interactions with different receptors displayed at the cell surface control a number of normal (e.g., lymphocyte activation and cell-cell adhesion) and abnormal (e.g., cell-pathogen adhesion and cancer cell metastasis) biological processes. Glycodendrimers have been synthesized by coupling isothiocyanate-functionalized glycosyl and mannopyranoside ligands as well as an *N*-hydroxysuccinimide (NHS)-activated galactopyranosyl derivative to amine-terminated dendrimers.

3.1.3. Hydrophobic dendrimers

Dendrimers with hydrophobic interiors and a hydrophilic surface are called hydrophobic dendrimers. Hydrophobic dendrimer gives better encapsulation and efficient solubilization of hydrophobic drug molecules. Specifically, dendrimers with hydrophobic cores were proved to effectively retain hydrophobic drug molecules in the voids of their branching architecture, mimicking amphiphilic polymer micelles.

3.1.4. *Asymmetric dendrimers*

Asymmetric dendrimers are synthesized by coupling dendrons of different generations to a linear core, which yields a branched dendrimer with a nonuniform orthogonal architecture.

There are two different types of dendrimeric copolymers:

1. **Segment-block dendrimers**—segmented with segments of different constitution.

2. **Layer-block dendrimers**—concentric spheres of differing chemistry [25–42].

4. Cationic polymers

DNA, when combined with sufficient amounts of cationic polymers, will condense into discrete entities which are called as polyplexes [43]. The polyplexes are compact nanoparticles formed through electrostatic interactions between the positive charges of amines and the negative charges of DNA phosphates. The strength of DNA binding to the polymers is related to the N:P ratio.

The most common cationic polymers used as nonviral gene-delivery vectors include chitosan, PLL, polyethylenimine (PEI), poly(amido amine) (PAMAM) dendrimers and select polypeptides [24, 44, 45].

4.1. Chitosan

Chitosan is a polysaccharide copolymer composed of randomly distributed β-(1-4)-linked d-glucosamines and *N*-acetyl-d-glucosamines, obtained by partial alkaline deacetylation of chitin [46], with different molecular weights (50–200 kDa), degrees of deacetylation (40–98%) and viscosities [47]. Chitosan is a natural polymer, **Figure 5**, with linear polyamine, having reactive amino and hydroxyl groups, biodegradable to normal body constituent, safe and non-toxic, and binds to mammalian and microbial cells. The main commercial sources of chitosan are the crustacean shell wastes of crabs, shrimps and

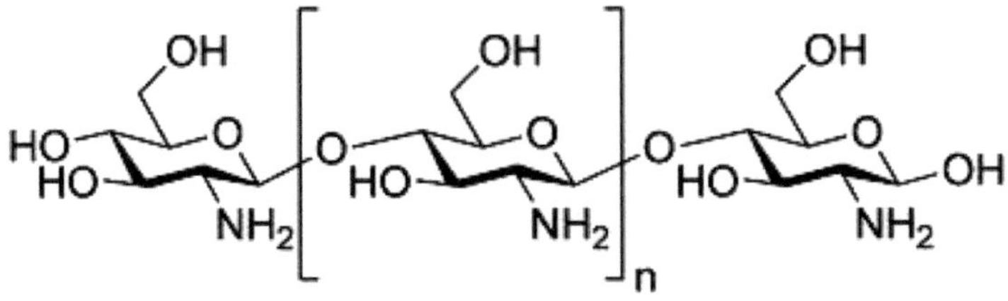

Figure 5. Structure of chitosan.

lobsters [48]. Chitosan is soluble in aqueous solutions of some acids and some selective N-alkylidination. Its solubility, biodegradability, reactivity and adsorptivity of many substrates depend on the amount of protonation of the $-NH_2$ function on the C-2 position of the D-glucosamine unit, whereby the polysaccharide is converted to a polyelectrolyte in acidic media. Chitosan is considered one of the most valuable polymers for biomedical and pharmaceutical applications due to its biodegradability, biocompatibility, antimicrobial, non-toxicity and anti-tumour properties.

Chitosan effectively condenses DNA and protects it from nuclease degradation. Various conjugates such as thiolation, glycolation and folate chitosan are available. Chitosan is biodegradable, biocompatible, low immunogenicity and non-toxic at low molecular weights (10–50 kDa). It has been suggested that the toxicity of chitosan is perhaps due to impurities in the chitosan polymers [49–60].

4.2. Poly-L-lysine

Poly-L-lysine (ε-poly-L-lysine), as given in **Figure 6**, is a small natural homopolymer of the essential amino acid L-lysine that is produced by bacterial fermentation. Poly-L-lysine is a positively charged amino acid polymer with approximately one HBr per lysine residue. The hydrobromide allows the poly-L-lysine to be in a crystalline form soluble in water. Adhesion

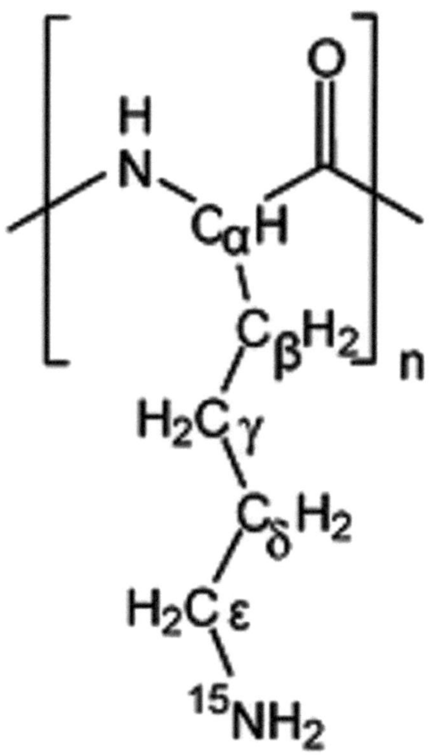

Figure 6. Structure of poly-L-lysine.

into the cell wall is based on the interaction between the negatively charged ions of the cell membrane and positive charge of poly-L-lysine. Simple electrostatic mixing of DNA and poly-L-lysine produces DNA particles with various structures. The mode of binding between the poly-L-lysine and DNA is cooperative and non-cooperative binding. Condensation between the DNA with the PLA depends upon the PLL chain length. Increase in the length of the PLL chain increases the condensation [61–68].

4.3. Polyethylenimine

Polyethylenimine (PEI), as given in **Figures 8** and **9**, is water-soluble, linear or branched polymers composed of the amine group and two carbon aliphatic CH_2CH_2 spacer. It is a weakly basic aliphatic polymer and polycationic one due to primary, secondary and tertiary amino groups. PEIs are available in different molecular masses and forms. Various forms of PEIs are shown in **Figure** 7–9. Linear polyethylenimines contain all secondary amines, whereas branched PEIs contain primary, secondary and tertiary amino groups. Due to their high cationic charge density at physiological pH, PEIs are able to form non-covalent complexes with DNA, siRNA and antisense oligodeoxynucleotide, and then brought into the cell via endocytosis. Once inside the cell, protonation of the amines results in an influx of counter-ions and a lowering of the osmotic potential, leading to bursts in the vesicle releasing the polymer-DNA complex (polyplex) into the cytoplasm. If the polyplex unpacks, then the DNA is free to diffuse to the nucleus; however, the long PEI chains have higher efficiency in gene transfection, and are more cytotoxic [69–93].

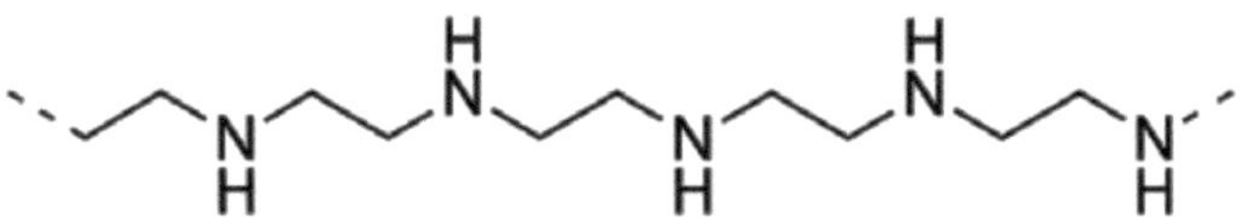

Figure 7. Structure of linear PEI.

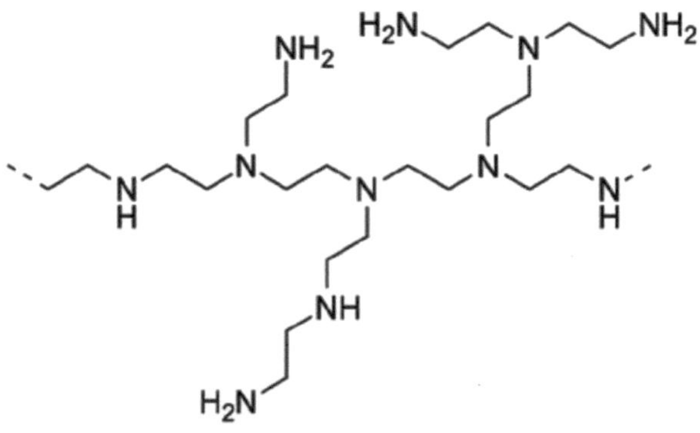

Figure 8. Structure of branched PEI.

http://dx.doi.org/10.5772/65694

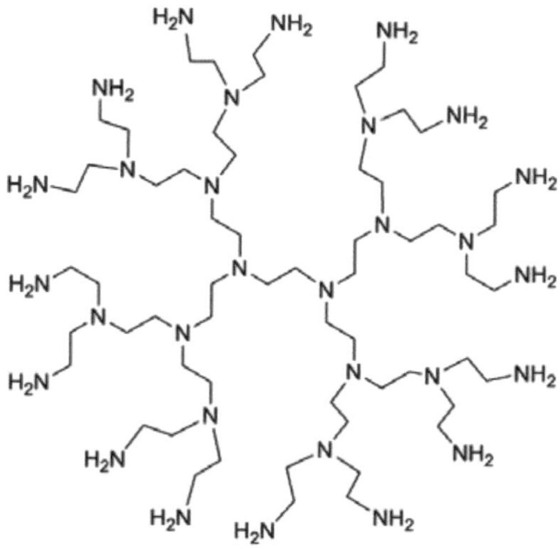

Figure 9. Structure of dendrimer PEI.

5. Cationic lipids

The four constituents are given as follows:

1. The cationic polar head group.
2. A hydrophobic chain that affects the physical properties of the lipid bilayer.
3. The space between two mentioned sections that improves chemical stability, biodegradability and gene transfection efficiency.
4. A backbone domain as a scaffold [19].

5.1. Monovalent cationic lipids

5.1.1. DOTMA

Chemically, it is N-[1-(2,3-dioleyloxy) propyl]-N,N,N-trimethylammonium chloride, as given in **Figure 10**, that consists of four different moieties: (1) a quaternary ammonium head group as the cationic head group, (2) a glycerol-based backbone, (3) two linkage bonds and (4) two hydrocarbon chains. Alternations can be made in the above moieties to reduce the toxicity and increase the gene transfection efficiencies. Replacement of a methyl group on the quaternary amine of DOTMA with a hydroxyl improves protein expression after gene transfection due to the replaced hydroxyl group in contact with the aqueous layer surrounding the liposome. Increase in the length of the aliphatic chain decreases the gene transfection and vice versa [94–98].

5.1.2. DOTAP

DOTAP, [1,2-bis(oleoyloxy)-3-(trimethylammonio) propane], as given in **Figure 11**, consists of a quaternary amine head group coupled to a glycerol backbone with two oleoyl chains.

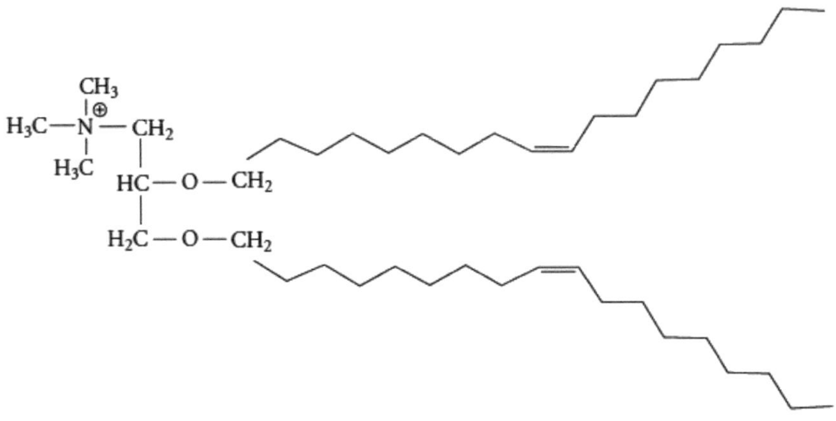

Figure 10. Structure of DOTMA.

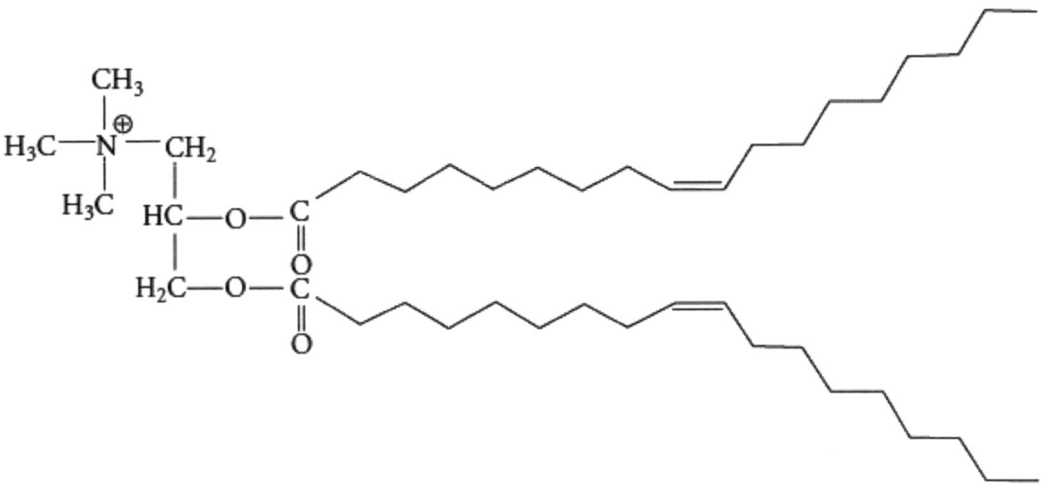

Figure 11. Structure of DOTAP.

The only differences between this molecule and DOTMA are that ester bonds link the chains to the backbone rather than ether bonds. The ester bonds present in the backbone are hydrolysable and lead to render the lipid biodegradable and reduce cytotoxicity. DOTAP cannot be used alone as a cationic liquid for gene delivery due to its dense positive charge, thereby preventing the ion exchange. Its gene-delivery efficiency can be changed by combining with other helper liquids [94, 99–103].

5.1.3. DC-Chol

3β[*N*-(*N′*,*N′*-dimethylaminoethane)-carbamoyl] cholesterol, as given in **Figure 12**, contains a cholesterol moiety attached by an ester bond to a hydrolysable dimethylethylenediamine. Due to the presence of cholesterol moiety, it is biocompatible and has good stability. The combination of DC-Chol and dioleoylphosphatidylethanolamine (DOPE) in the ratio 1:1

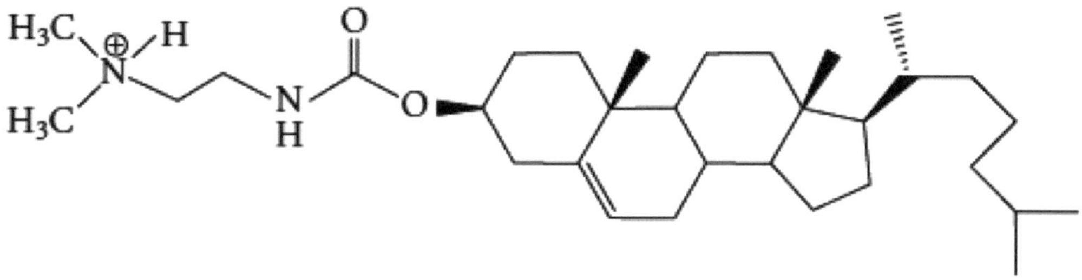

Figure 12. Structure of DC-Col.

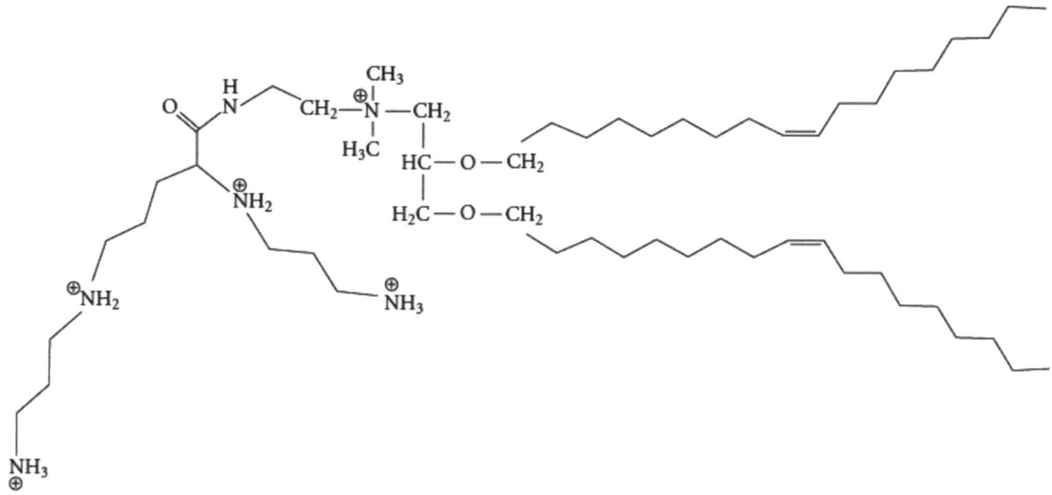

Figure 13. Structure of DOSPA.

reduces the lipoplex aggregation; it assists the DNA dissociation during gene delivery [94, 99, 100, 103, 104].

5.2. Multivalent cationic lipids

5.2.1. DOSPA

DOSPA is a derivative of DOTMA. Chemically, it is 2,3-dioleyloxy-N-[2(sperminecarboxamido) ethyl]-N,N-dimethyl-l-propanaminium trifluoroacetate, which is given in **Figure 13**. The difference between DOSPA and DOTMA is a spermine group, which is bound through a peptide bond to the hydrophobic chains. Spermine group allows more efficient packing of DNA due to its hydrogen bond interaction with the DNA [43, 94].

5.2.2. DOGS

DOGS, chemically it is di-octadecyl-amido-glycyl-spermine, structure of the DOGS is similar to DOSPA, as given in **Figure 14**. The molecular structures of both DOGS and DOSPA consist of a multivalent spermine head group and two 18-carbon alkyl chains. The saturated chains

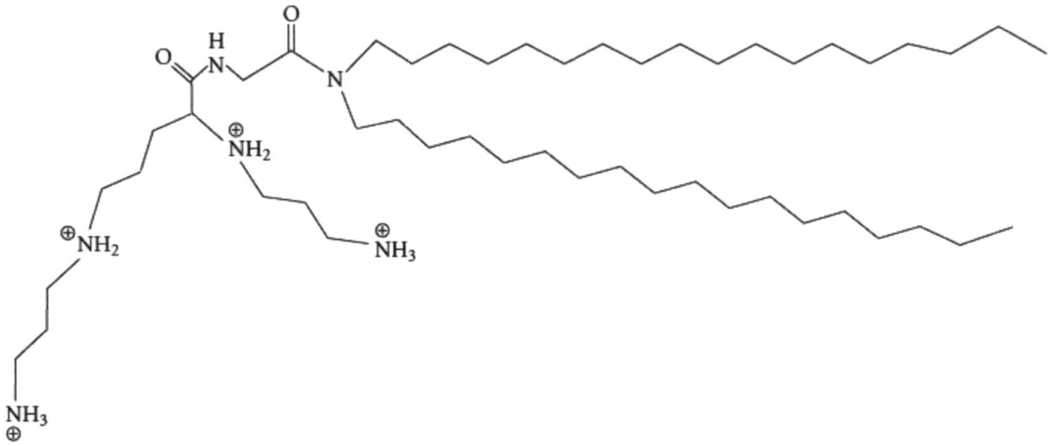

Figure 14. Structure of DOGS.

in DOGS are linked to the head group through a peptide bond. The packing ability of DNA by DOGS is due to its large head group molecule and the length of long unsaturated carbon chains. DOGS have efficient packing of DNA, due to its spermine head group. The presence of spermine head group in DOGS leads to efficient packing of DNA [94, 105–107].

6. Neutral lipids

The commonly used neutral lipids are dioleoylphosphatidylethanolamine (DOPE), as given in **Figure 15**, and dioleoylphosphatidylcholine (DOPC), as given in **Figure 16**. These neutral lipids are used in combination with the other cationic polymers. The gene transfection efficiencies of the cationic polymer are increased when it is used in combination with the helper neutral liquids. The increase in gene transfection efficiency is due to conformational shift to an inverted hexagonal packing structure like a honeycomb by DOPE at lower or acidic pH. The formation

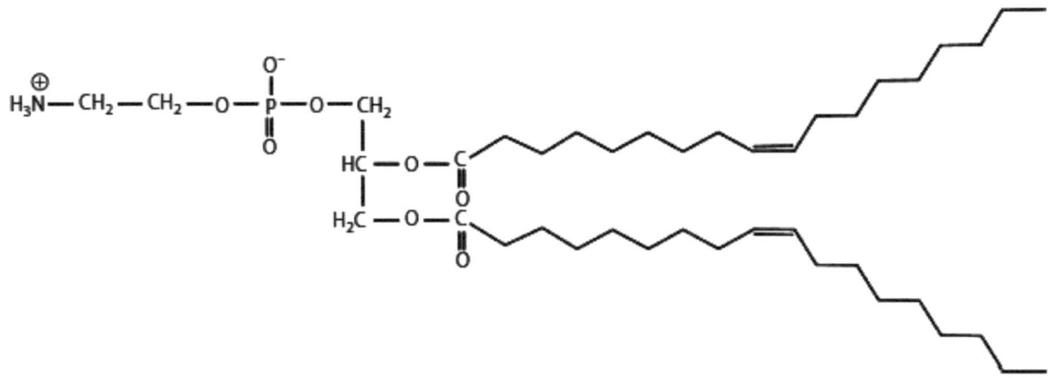

Figure 15. Structure of DOPE.

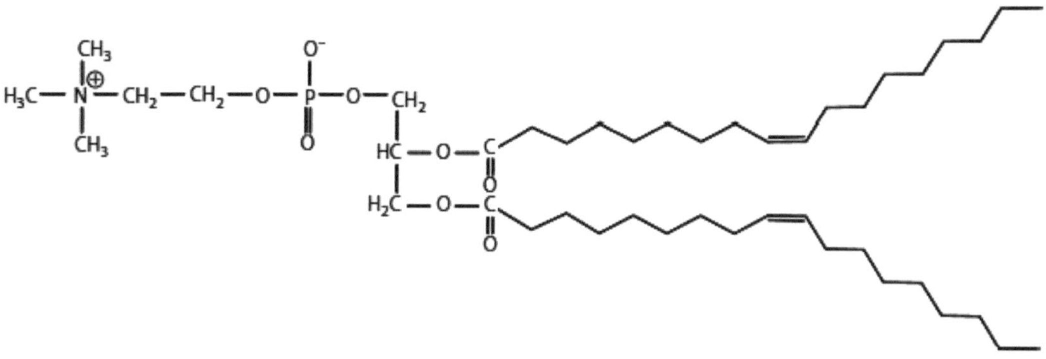

Figure 16. Structure of DOPC.

of inverted hexagonal-packing structure condenses the DNA inside by electrostatic interactions. During gene transfection, fusion and destabilization of the lipoplex occur which lead to the release of DNA from endosomal vesicles. Cationic polymers DOTAP, DC-Chol and other cholesterol derivatives have been incorporated with DOPE for gene transfection efficiency [94, 103, 108–114].

7. Poly(ethylene) glycol (PEG)

Chemically, poly(ethylene) glycol (PEG) ($C_{2n}H_{4n+2}O_{n+1}$) is a polyether or polymer of ethylene oxide.

The physical properties of PEG vary with respect to its chain length, whereas its chemical properties are almost the same. It is available in different molecular weights and different geometries such as branched PEG, star PEG and comb PEG. PEG is non-toxic and excreted through kidney. Degradation of the drug can be protected due to its surface modification property, and it has been extensively used as liposomal targeting by liposomal coating. The liposomes have longer circulation time in blood, reduced macrophage uptake, higher gene transfection efficiencies, larger available concentration and bioavailability [94, 115–120].

8. Conclusion

Nanotechnology is a science adapted in various research areas specifically in the drug-delivery system. At present, gene delivery system includes viral-based, non-viral-based and combined hybrid systems, which are widely used for the treatment of various diseases. To provide the desired concentration of the drug in the target site and therapeutic effect is critical of the drug-delivery system. Biopolymer is a biomaterial that has been utilized extensively for formulating genetic material into a nanoparticle either embedded or encapsulated within the polymeric matrix. Despite various biopolymers, choosing a suitable biopolymer, nanoparticle preparation procedure with desired properties can achieve the bio-distribution and effective delivery of the genetic material into the target site and regulate the damaged genes to produce the required proteins.

Author details

Sakthivel Lakshmana Prabu[1*] and Kandasamy Ruckmani[1,2]

*Address all correspondence to: slaxmanvel@gmail.com

1 Department of Pharmaceutical Technology, Bharathidasan Institute of Technology, Anna University, Tiruchirapalli, Tamil Nadu, India

2 Centre for Excellence in Nanobio Translational Research (CENTRE), National Facility on Drug Design (NFDD), Professor and Head, Department of Pharmaceutical Technology, Bharathidasan Institute of Technology, Anna University, Tiruchirapalli, Tamil Nadu, India

References

[1] Ward MA, Georgiou TK. Thermoresponsive polymers for biomedical applications. Polymers. 2011; 3: 1215–1242.

[2] Twaites BR, Alarcon CDH, Lavigne M, Saulnier A, Pennadam SS, Cunliffe D, et al., Thermoresponsive polymers as gene delivery vectors: Cell viability, DNA transport and transfection studies. J Control Release. 2005; 108: 472–473.

[3] Mahapatra A, Singh DK. Biodegradable nanoparticle are excellent vehicle for site directed in-vivo delivery of drugs and vaccines. J Nanobiotech. 2011; 9: 55.

[4] Mishra B, Vuppu S, Rath K. The role of microbial pullulan, a biopolymer in pharmaceutical approaches: A review. J Appl Pharm Sci. 2011; 1(6): 45–50.

[5] Eliyahu H, Barenholz Y, Domb AJ. Polymers for DNA delivery. Molecules. 2005; 10: 34–64.

[6] Pack DW, Hoffman AS, Pun S, Stayton PS. Design and development of polymers for gene delivery. Nature Rev Drug Discov. 2005; 4: 581–593.

[7] Dang JM, Leong KW. Natural polymers for gene delivery and tissue engineering. Adv Drug Del Rev. 2006; 58(4): 487–499.

[8] Nitta SK, Numata K. Biopolymer based nanoparticles for drug/gene delivery and tissue engineering. Int J Mol Sci. 2013; 14: 1629–1654.

[9] Harris TJ, Green JJ, Fung PW, Langer R, Anderson DG, Bhatia SN. Tissue specific gene delivery via nanoparticle coating. Biomaterials. 2010; 31(5): 998–1006.

[10] Labhasetwar V, Song C, Levy RJ. Nanoparticle drug delivery system for restenosis. Adv Drug Del Rev. 1997; 24(1): 63–85.

[11] Erdal C, Ali DS, Emre SC. Gene delivery systems: Recent progress in viral and non-viral therapy. In: Recent Advances in Novel Drug Carrier Systems, Ali DS (Ed.), 2012, InTech, Croatia, DOI: 10.5772/53392. http://www.intechopen.com/books/recent-advances-in-novel-drug-carrier-systems/gene-delivery-systems-recent-progress-in-viral-and-non-viral-therapy

[12] Liang GF, Zhu YL, Sun B, Hu FH, Tian T, Li SC, et al. PLGA-based gene delivering nanoparticle enhance suppression effect of miRNA in HePG2 cells. Nanoscale Res Lett. 2011; 6: 447.

[13] Jin S, Ye K. Mediated drug delivery and gene therapy. Biotechnol Prog. 2007; 23: 32–41.

[14] Georgiou TK, Vamvakaki M, Patrickios CS, Yamasaki EN, Phylactou LA. Nanoscopic cationic methacrylate star homopolymers: Synthesis by group transfer polymerization, characterization and evaluation as transfection reagents. Biomacromolecules. 2004; 5 (6):2221–2229.

[15] Godbey WT. Mikos AG. Recent progress in gene delivery using non-viral transfer complexes. J Cont Release. 2001; 72 (1–3):115–125.

[16] Xu FJ, Zhang ZX, Ping Y, Li J, Kang ET, Neoh KG. Star-shaped cationic polymers by atom transfer radical polymerization from beta-cyclodextrin cores for nonviral gene delivery. Biomacromolecules. 2009; 10 (2):285–293.

[17] Cloninger MJ. Biological applications of dendrimers. Curr Opin Chem Biol. 2002; 6 (6):742–748.

[18] Tang MX, Redemann CT, Szoka C. *In vitro* gene delivery by degraded polyamidoamine dendrimers. Bioconjug Chem. 1996; 7 (6):703–714.

[19] Dizaj SM, Jafari S, Khosroushahi AY. A sight on the current nanoparticle-based gene delivery vectors. Nanoscale Res Lett. 2014; 9: 252.

[20] Kabanov AV, Kabanov VA. DNA complexes with polycations for the delivery of genetic material into cells. Bioconjug Chem. 1995; 6: 7–20.

[21] Ledley FD. Pharmaceutical approach to somatic gene therapy. Pharm Res. 1996; 13: 1595–1614.

[22] Vijayanatham V, Thomas T, Thomas TJ. DNA nanoparticles and development of DNA delivery vehicles for gene therapy. Biochemistry. 2002; 41:14085–14094.

[23] Armstrong, TKC, Girouard LG, Anchordoquy TJ. Effects of PEGylation on preservation of cationic lipid/DNA complexes during freeze-thawing and lyophilization. J Pharm Sci. 2002; 91:2549–2558.

[24] Oyewumi MO, Rice KG. DNA nanoparticle gene delivery systems. In: Nanoparticle Technology for Drug Delivery. Gupta RB, Kompella UB (eds.). Marcel Dekker, New York, Vol. 159, 2006; pp. 361–379.

[25] Boas U, Heegaard PM. Dendrimers in drug research. Chem Soc Rev. 2004; 33: 43–63.

[26] Cheng Y, Wang J, Rao T, He X, Xu, T. Pharmaceutical applications of dendrimers: Promising nanocarriers for drug delivery. Front Biosci. 2008; 13: 1447–1471.

[27] Dufes C, Uchegbu IF, Schatzlein AG. Dendrimers in gene delivery. Adv Drug Deliv Rev. 2005; 57; 2177–2202.

[28] Gao Y, Gao G, He Y, Liu T, Qi R. Recent advances of dendrimers in delivery of genes and drugs. Mini Rev Med Chem. 2008; 8: 889–900.

[29] Gillies ER, Frechet JM. Dendrimers and dendritic polymers in drug delivery. Drug Discov Today. 2005; 10: 35–43.

[30] Svenson S, Tomalia DA. Dendrimers in biomedical applications--reflections on the field. Adv Drug Deliv Rev. 2005; 57: 2106–2129.

[31] Tomalia DA, Baker H, Dewald J, Hall M, Kallos G, Martin S, et al. Dendritic macromolecules: Synthesis of starburst dendrimers. Macromolecules. 1986, 19: 2466–2468.

[32] Klajnert B, Bryszewska M. Dendrimers: Properties and applications. Acta Biochem Polonica. 2001; 48: 199–208.

[33] Tomalia DA, Baker H, Dewald JR, Hall M, Kallos G, Martin S, Roeck J, Ryder, J., Smith P. A new class of polymers: Starburst-dendritic macromolecules. Polym J. 1985; 17: 117–132.

[34] Fischer M, Vogtle F. Dendrimers: From design to applications—A progress report. Angew Chem Int Ed. 1999; 38: 884–905.

[35] Zimmerman SC, Zeng F, Reichert DEC, Kolotuchin SV. Self-assembling dendrimers. Science. 1996; 271: 1095–1098.

[36] Frechet JMJ. Functional polymers and dendrimers: Reactivity, molecular architecture, and interfacial energy. Science. 1994; 263: 1710–1715.

[37] Tomalia DA, Dvornic PR. What promise for dendrimers? Nature. 1994; 372: 617–618.

[38] Twyman LJ, Beezer AE, Esfand R, Hardy MJ, Mitchell JC. The synthesis of water soluble dendrimers, and their application as possible drug delivery systems. Tetrahedron Lett. 1999; 40: 1743–1746.

[39] Waite CL, Sparks SM, Uhrich KE, Roth CM. Acetylation of pamam dendrimers for cellular delivery of sirna. BMC Biotechnol. 2009; 9: 38.

[40] Biswas S, Vladimir P. Torchilin. Dendrimers for siRNA delivery. Pharmaceuticals. 2013; 6: 161–183.

[41] Medina SH, El-Sayed MEH. Dendrimers as carriers for delivery of chemotherapeutic agents. Chem Rev. 2009; 109: 3141–3157.

[42] Tomalia DA, Frechet JMJ. Discovery of dendrimers and dendritic polymers: A brief historical perspective. J Polym Sci Part A: Polym Chem. 2002; 40(16): 2719–2728.

[43] Vuorimaa E, Urtti A, Seppänen R, Lemmetyinen H, Yliperttula M. Time-resolved fluorescence spectroscopy reveals functional differences of cationic polymer-DNA complexes. J Am Chem Soc. 2008; 130(35): 11695–11700.

[44] Guo P, Coban O, Snead NM, Trebley J, Hoeprich S, Guo S, et al. Engineering RNA for targeted siRNA delivery and medical application. Adv Drug Deliv Rev. 2010; 62: 650–666.

[45] Nimesh S, Gupta N, Chandra R. Cationic polymer based nanocarriers for delivery of therapeutic nucleic acids. J Biomed Nanotechnol. 2011; 7: 504–520.

[46] Synowiecki J, Al-Khateeb NA. Production, properties, and some new applications of chitin and its derivatives. Crit Rev Food Sci Nutr. 2003; 43(2): 145–171.

[47] Illum L. Chitosan and its use as a pharmaceutical excipient. Pharm Res. 1998; 15(9): 1326–1331.

[48] Hggard MK, Tubulekas I, Guan H, Edwards K, Nilsson M, Varum KM, et al., Chitosan as a nonviral gene delivery system. Structure property relationships and characteristics compared with polyethylenimine in vitro and after lung administration in vivo. Gene Ther. 2001; 8(14): 1108–1121.

[49] Lee M, Nah JW, Kwon Y, Koh JJ, Ko KS, Kim SW. Water-soluble and low molecular weight chitosan-based plasmid DNA delivery. Pharm Res. 2001; 18(4): 427–431.

[50] Lee D, Zhang W, Shirley SA, Kong X, Hellermann GR, Lockey RF, et al. Thiolated chitosan/DNA nanocomplexes exhibit enhanced and sustained gene delivery. Pharm Res. 2007; 24(1): 157–167.

[51] Mathur NK, Narang CK. Chitin and chitosan, versatile polysaccharides from marine animals. J Chem Educ. 1990; 67:938–42.

[52] Hudson SM, Jenkins DW. Chitin and chitosan. In: Encyclopedia of Polymer Science and Technology. Mark HF (ed.), New York, NY: Wiley; 2003. pp. 569–80.

[53] Krajewska B. Application of chitin- and chitosan-based materials for enzyme immobilizations: A review. Enzyme Microbiol Technol. 2004; 35: 126–139.

[54] Kanke M, Katayama H, Tsuzuki S, Kuramoto H. Application of chitin and chitosan to pharmaceutical preparations. Chem Pharm Bull. 1989; 37: 523–25.

[55] Kato Y, Onishi H, Machida Y. Application of chitin and chitosan derivatives in the pharmaceutical field. Curr Pharm Biotechnol. 2003; 4: 303–309.

[56] Anthonsen MW, Varum KM, Smidsrod O. Solution properties of chitosans: Conformation and chain stiffness of chitosans with different degrees of N-acetylation. Carbohyd Polym. 1993; 22: 193–201.

[57] Rinaudo M. Chitin and chitosan: Properties and applications. Prog Polym Sci. 2006; 31: 603–632.

[58] Alvarenga ES. Characterization and properties of chitosan. In: Biotechnology of Biopolymers. Elnashar M (ed.), InTech. 2011; pp. 91–108.

[59] Tungtong S, Okonogi S, Chowwanapoonpohn S, Phutdhawong W, Yotsawimonwat S. Solubility, viscosity and rheological properties of water-soluble chitosan derivatives. Maejo Int J Sci Technol. 2012; 6(2): 315–322.

[60] Pillai CKS, Paul W, Sharma CP. Chitin and chitosan polymers: Chemistry, solubility and fiber formation. Prog Polym Sci. 2009; 34: 641–678.

[61] Laemmli UK. Characterization of DNA condensates induced by poly(ethylene oxide) and polylysine. Proc Nat Acad Sci USA. 1975; 72(11): 4288–4292.

[62] Gonsho A, Irie K, Susaki H, Iwasawa H, Okuno S, Sugawara T. Tissue-targeting ability of saccharide-poly(L-lysine) conjugates. Biol Pharm Bull. 1994; 17(2): 275–282.

[63] Shima S, Sakai H. Polylysine produced by Streptomyces. Agric Biol Chem. 1977; 41: 1807–1809.

[64] Liu G, Molas M, Grossmann GA, Pasumarthy M, Perales JC, Cooper MJ, et al. Biological properties of poly-L-lysine-DNA complexes generated by cooperative binding of the polycation. J Biol Chem. 2001; 276(37): 34379–34387.

[65] Ferdous A, Watanabe H, Akaike T, Maruyama A. Comb-type copolymer: Stabilization of triplex DNA and possible application in antigene strategy. J Pharm Sci. 1998; 87(11): 1400–1405.

[66] Krikorian V, Kurian M, Galvin ME, Nowak AP, Deming TJ, Pochan DJ. Polypeptide-based nanocomposite: Structure and properties of poly(L-lysine)/Na_-montmorillonite. J Poly. Sci Part B: Poly Phys. 2002; 40: 2579–2586.

[67] Liu G, Molas M, Grossmann GA, Pasumarthy M, Perales JC, Cooper MJ, et al. Binding of the polycation complexes generated by cooperative biological properties of poly-l-lysine-DNA. J Biol Chem. 2001; 276: 34379–34387.

[68] Toncheva V, Wolfert MA, Dash PR, Oupicky D, Ulbrich K, Seymour LW, Schacht EH. Novel vectors for gene delivery formed by self-assembly of DNA with poly(L-lysine) grafted with hydrophilic polymers. Biochim Biophys Acta. 1998; 1380: 354–368.

[69] Boussif O, Zanta MA, Behr JP. Optimized galenics improve in vitro gene transfer with cationic molecules up to 1000-fold. Gene Ther. 1996; 3(12): 1074–1080.

[70] Godbey WT, Barry MA, Saggau P, Wu KK, Mikos AG. Poly(ethylenimine)-mediated transfection: A new paradigm for gene delivery. J Biomed Mater Res. 2000; 51(3): 321–328.

[71] Yao YH, Liu YB, Feng Y, Feng X, Xu DM, Yao SD. Synthesis and screening of polyethylenimine as a carrier for gene transfer into cultured human tumor cells. Ai Zheng. 2007; 26(7): 790–794.

[72] Sharma VK, Thomas M, Klibanov AM. Mechanistic studies on aggregation of polyethylenimine-DNA complexes and its prevention. Biotechnol Bioeng. 2005; 90(5): 614–620.

[73] Ogris M, Steinlein P, Kursa M, Mechtler K, Kircheis R, Wagner E. The size of DNA/transferrin-PEI complexes is an important factor for gene expression in cultured cells. Gene Ther. 1998; 5(10): 1425–1433.

[74] Lee H, Jeong JH, Park TG. A new gene delivery formulation of polyethylenimine/DNA complexes coated with PEG conjugated fusogenic peptide. J Con Rel. 2001; 76(1–2): 183–192.

[75] Aoki K, Furuhata S, Hatanaka K, Maeda M, Remy JS, Behr JP, et al. Polyethylenimine-mediated gene transfer into pancreatic tumor dissemination in the murine peritoneal cavity. Gene Ther. 2001; 8: 508–514.

[76] Boussif O, Lezoualc'h F, Zanta MA, Mergny MD, Scherman D, Demeneix B, et al. A versatile vector for gene and oligonucleotide transfer into cells in culture and in vivo: Polyethylenimine. Proc Natl Acad Sci USA. 1995; 92: 7297–7301.

[77] Lungwitz U, Breunig M, Blunk T, Gopferich A. Polyethylenimine-based non-viral gene delivery systems. Eur J Pharm Biopharm. 2005; 60: 247–266.

[78] Zintchenko A, Philipp A, Dehshahri A, Wagner E. Simple modifications of branched PEI lead to highly efficient sirna carriers with low toxicity. Bioconjug Chem. 2008; 19: 1448–1455.

[79] Lee M, Kim SW. Polyethylene glycol-conjugated copolymers for plasmid DNA delivery. Pharm Res. 2005; 22: 1–10.

[80] Nimesh S. Polyethylenimine as a promising vector for targeted sirna delivery. Curr Clin Pharmacol. 2012; 7: 121–130.

[81] Petersen H, Fechner PM, Martin AL, Kunath K, Stolnik S, Roberts CJ, Fischer D, Davies MC, Kissel T. Polyethylenimine-graft-poly(ethylene glycol) copolymers: Influence of copolymer block structure on DNA complexation and biological activities as gene delivery system. Bioconjug Chem. 2002; 13(4): 845–854.

[82] Godbey WT, Wu KK, Mikos AG: Poly (ethylenimine)-mediated gene delivery affects endothelial cell function and viability. Biomaterials. 2000; 22: 471–480.

[83] Godbey WT, Wu KK, Mikos AG. Size matters: Molecular weight affects the efficiency of poly(ethylenimine) as a gene delivery vehicle. J Biomed Mater Res. 1999; 45: 268–275.

[84] Fischer D, Bieber T, Li Y, Elsässer HP, Kissel T. A novel non-viral vector for DNA delivery based on low molecular weight, branched polyethylenimine: Effect of molecular weigh on transfection efficiency and cytotoxicity. Pharm Res. 1999; 16:1273–1279.

[85] Furgeson DY, Chan WS, Yockman JW, Kim SW. Modified linear polyethylenimine-cholesterol conjugates for DNA complexation. Bioconjugate Chem. 2003; 14: 840–847.

[86] Furgeson DY, Yockman JW, Janat MM, Kim SW: Tumor efficacy and biodistribution of linear polyethylenimine-cholesterol/DNA complexes. Mol Ther. 2004; 9: 837–845.

[87] Thomas M, Lu J, Ge Q, Zhang C, Chen J, Klibanov AM. Full deacylation of polyethylenimine dramatically boosts its gene delivery efficiency and specificity to mouse lung. Proc Natl Acad Sci USA. 2005; 102: 5679–5684.

[88] Jeon O, Yang HS, Lee TJ, Kim BS. Heparin-conjugated polyethylenimine for gene delivery. J Control Release. 2008; 132: 236–242.

[89] Xu Z, Shen G, Xia X, Zhao X, Zhang P, Wu H, et al. Comparisons of three polyethylenimine-derived nanoparticles as a gene therapy delivery system for renal cell carcinoma. J Transl Med. 2011; 9: 46.

[90] Felt O, Buri P, Guruy R. Chitosan: A unique polysaccharide for drug delivery. Drug Dev Ind Pharm. 1998; 24: 979.

[91] Tang MX, Szoka FC. The influence of polymer structure on the interactions of cationic polymers with DNA and morphology of the resulting complexes. Gene Ther. 1997; 4: 823–832.

[92] Fischer D, Bieber T, Li YX, Elsasser HP, Kissel T. A novel non-viral vector for DNA delivery based on low molecular weight, branched polyethylenimine: Effect of molecular weight on transfection efficiency and cytotoxicity. Pharm Res. 1999; 16: 1273–79.

[93] Von Harpe A, Petersen H, Li YX, Kissel T. Characterization of commercially available and synthesized polyethylenimines for gene delivery. J Control Release. 2000; 69: 309–322.

[94] Zhang X, Balazs DA, Godbey WT. Nanobiomaterials for nonviral gene delivery. In: Nanobiomaterials Hand Book, Balaji Sitharaman (ed.). CRC press, Taylor & Francis, 2011, pp.13–1 to 13–25.

[95] Ren T, Song YK, Zhang G, Liu D. Structural basis of DOTMA for its high intravenous transfection activity in mouse. Gene Therapy. 2000; 7: 764–768.

[96] Leventis R, Silvius JR. Interactions of mammalian cells with lipid dispersions containing novel metabolizable cationic amphiphiles. Biochim Biophys Acta. 1990; 1023: 124–32.

[97] Gao X, Huang L. A novel cationic liposome reagent for efficient transfection of mammalian cells. Biochem Biophys Res Commun. 1991; 179: 280–285.

[98] Malone RW, Felgner PL, Verma IM. Cationic liposome-mediated RNA transfection. Proc Natl Acad Sci USA. 1989; 86: 6077–6081.

[99] Zuidam NJ, Barenholz Y. Electrostatic and structural properties of complexes involving plasmid DNA and cationic lipids commonly used for gene delivery. Biochim Biophys Acta. 1998; 1368: 115–128.

[100] Zabner J, Fasbender AJ, Moninger T, Poellinger KA, Welsh MJ. Cellular and molecular barriers to gene transfer by a cationic lipid. J Biol Chem. 1995; 270: 18997–9007.

[101] Yang JP, Huang L. Time-dependent maturation of cationic liposome-DNA complex for serum resistance. Gene Ther.1998; 5: 380–387.

[102] Marchini C, Montani M, Amici M, Amenitsch H, Marianecci C, Pozzi D, et al. Structural stability and increase in size rationalize the efficiency of lipoplexes in serum. Langmuir. 2009; 25: 3013–3021.

[103] Gao X, Huang L. A novel cationic liposome reagent for efficient transfection of mammalian cells. Biochem Biophys Res Commun. 1991; 179(1): 280–285.

[104] Zuidam NJ, Barenholz Y. Electrostatic parameters of cationic liposomes commonly used for gene delivery as determined by 4-heptadecyl-7-hydroxycoumarin. Biochim Biophys Acta. 1997; 1329(2): 211–222.

[105] Behr JP, Demeneix B, Loeffler JP, Perez-Mutul J. Efficient gene transfer into mammalian primary endocrine cells with lipopolyamine-coated DNA. Proc Natl Acad Sci USA. 1989; 86(18): 6982–6986.

[106] Boukhnikachvili T, Aguerre-Chariol O, Airiau M, Lesieur S, Ollivon M, Vacus J. Structure of in-serum transfecting DNA-cationic lipid complexes. FEBS Lett. 1997; 409(2): 188–194.

[107] Remy JS, Sirlin C, Vierling P, Behr JP. Gene transfer with a series of lipophilic DNA-binding molecules. Bioconjug Chem. 1994; 5(6): 647–654.

[108] Farhood H, Gao X, Son K, Yang YY, Lazo JS, Huang L, et al. Cationic liposomes for direct gene transfer in therapy of cancer and other diseases. Ann N Y Acad Sci. 1994; 716: 23–34.

[109] Farhood H, Serbina N, Huang L. The role of dioleoyl phosphatidylethanolamine in cationic liposome mediated gene transfer. Biochim Biophys Acta. 1995; 1235(2): 289–295.

[110] Chesnoy S, Huang L. Structure and function of lipid-DNA complexes for gene delivery. Annu Rev Biophys Biomol Struct. 2000; 29: 27–47.

[111] Hui SW, Langner M, Zhao YL, Ross P, Hurley E, Cha K. The role of helper lipids in cationic liposome-mediated gene transfer. Biophys J. 1996; 71(2): 590–599.

[112] Kawakami S, Yamashita F, Nishikawa M, Takakura Y, Hashida M. Asialoglycoprotein receptor-mediated gene transfer using novel galactosylated cationic liposomes. Biochem Biophys Res Commun. 1998; 252(1): 78–83.

[113] Legendre JY, Szoka Jr FC. Delivery of plasmid DNA into mammalian cell lines using pH-sensitive liposomes: Comparison with cationic liposomes. Pharm Res. 1992; 9(10): 1235–1242.

[114] Zuhorn IS, Bakowsky U, Polushkin E, Visser WH, Stuart MC, Engberts JB, Hoekstra D. Nonbilayer phase of lipoplex-membrane mixture determines endosomal escape of genetic cargo and transfection efficiency. Mol Ther. 2005; 11(5): 801–810.

[115] Decastro M, Saijoh Y, Schoenwolf GC. Optimized cationic lipid-based gene delivery reagents for use in developing vertebrate embryos. Dev Dyn. 2006; 235(8): 2210–2219.

[116] Ishida O, Maruyama K, Tanahashi H, Iwatsuru M, Sasaki K, Eriguchi M, et al., Liposomes bearing polyethyleneglycol-coupled transferrin with intracellular targeting property to the solid tumors in vivo. Pharm Res. 2001; 18(7): 1042–1048.

[117] Huang RQ, Qu YH, Ke WL, Zhu JH, Pei YY, Jiang C. Efficient gene delivery targeted to the brain using a transferrin conjugated polyethyleneglycol-modified polyamidoamine dendrimer. FASEB J. 2007; 21(4): 1117–1125.

[118] Kim JK, Choi SH, Kim CO, Park JS, Ahn WS, Kim CK. Enhancement of polyethylene glycol (PEG)-modified cationic liposome-mediated gene deliveries: Effects on serum stability and transfection efficiency. J Pharm Pharmacol. 2003; 55(4): 453–460.

[119] Kim TI, Seo HJ, Choi JS, Jang HS, Baek JU, Kim K, et al. PAMAM-PEG-PAMAM: Novel triblock copolymer as a biocompatible and efficient gene delivery carrier. Biomacromolecules. 2004; 5(6): 2487–2492.

[120] Metselaar JM, Bruin P, de Boer LW, de Vringer T, Snel C, Oussoren C, et al. A novel family of L-amino acid-based biodegradable polymer-lipid conjugates for the development of long-circulating liposomes with effective drug-targeting capacity. Bioconjug Chem. 2003; 14(6): 1156–1164.

Chapter 8

Nuclear Medicine and Drug Delivery

Ana Rita Fernandes, Ana Oliveira, Jorge Pereira and
Pedro Silva Coelho

Additional information is available at the end of the chapter

http://dx.doi.org/10.5772/65708

Abstract

Nuclear Medicine is a molecular-imaging modality that diagnoses and treats diseases with very small amounts of radioactive materials, known as radiopharmaceuticals. Drug delivery refers to approaches, formulations, technologies, and systems for transporting a pharmaceutical compound in the body as needed to safely achieve its desired therapeutic effect. The use of nuclear medicine and radiopharmaceuticals allows studying the *in vivo* behavior of developed drug-delivery systems, and pharmacoscintigraphy is, from the beginning, one of the most promising aspects of this medical specialty. In this chapter, we review the technologies, fundaments, rationales, and strategies more frequently used and present examples of their application in the development and evaluation of drug-delivery systems.

Keywords: nuclear medicine, radiopharmaceuticals, drug delivery, *in vivo* analysis

1. Introduction

Nuclear Medicine is a medical speciality that involves the application of small amounts of radioactive materials, known as radiopharmaceuticals, for the diagnosis and treatment of disease, without causing any physiological effect.

Drug-delivery strategies have been steadily being developed in order to obtain better therapeutic results, enhance adhesion to treatment, and mitigate side effects. The ever-increasing complexity of the systems, combined with the regulatory demands by the Medicines Authorities, made the *in vivo* analysis of those systems' behavior almost compulsory.

The unique characteristics of Nuclear Medicine and Radiopharmaceuticals make dynamic, noninvasive studies and therefore are frequently used in the evaluation and development of new drug-delivery systems. This chapter aims to review the different techniques available, their rationale and applications, using, whenever possible, examples from the literature as well as from the authors' own experience.

2. Molecular imaging and Nuclear Medicine

Molecular imaging is defined as the visualization, characterization, and measurement of physiological mechanisms at the molecular and cellular levels, in living systems. Apart from Nuclear Medicine, it includes several other techniques, such as magnetic resonance imaging and spectroscopy, certain ultrasound technologies, and others [1, 2].

One of the biggest advantages of molecular imaging is the ability to characterize specific disease processes in different individuals, using noninvasive assessment and quantification; i.e., providing information that is inaccessible with any other imaging techniques or that otherwise would require more invasive procedures such as biopsy or surgery. Also, it identifies disease in its earliest phases and determines the precise location of a tumor, frequently before symptoms occur or changes can be detected at the anatomical level. Identifying small differences between patients allows the tailoring of specific treatments for each individual [1–3].

Nuclear Medicine is a molecular-imaging modality that diagnoses and treats diseases using radioactive materials, known as radiopharmaceuticals. Radiopharmaceuticals, at diagnostic levels, have the ability to portray human physiology, biochemistry, or pathology without causing any physiological effect [1, 3].

For example, it can be used to identify the presence or absence of specific receptors or molecular changes, which are crucial for the selection of patients for certain targeted therapies [1].

This step for "personalized medicine" also allows a more precise identification of research subjects, leading to more exact and cost-effective clinical trials [3].

3. Detectors and imaging systems

Diagnostic imaging refers to the techniques and processes used to create anatomical and functional images and is one of the fields in Medicine with the greater recent development [1].

The first reference to structural imaging dates to 1895, when Wilhelm Conrad Röntgen identified electromagnetic radiation in a wavelength range now known as X-rays. Functional imaging started following the discovery of the scintillation scanner by Benedict Casen (using I-131 as a radiotracer for diagnostic imaging purpose), and developed as a diagnostic specialty in 1958, when Hal Anger introduced the gamma camera (based on the principle of scintillation counting). Since then, Nuclear Medicine has considerably changed our view of looking at disease, by showing images of radiotracer distributions, providing functional images [1, 4].

A gamma camera is single-photon imaging equipment, also known as Anger camera or as scintillation camera. It contains a large radiation detector, consisting of a large thallium-activated sodium iodide crystal—the scintillator. A collimator, placed in front of the crystal, enables the γ-rays to be focused onto the detector. Coupled to the crystal are photomultiplier tubes, which detect the light pulses. The whole detection part of the equipment is shielded from undesirable radiation. An electronic system links the photomultiplier tubes to a computer and visual display unit [1, 5, 6, 7].

The basic principle of gamma cameras is that radionuclide concentrations in the body can be measured *in vivo*, by detecting the photons emitted during their radioactive decay. The first gamma cameras were only able to create two-dimensional (2D) representations. But in 1963, David Kuhl and Roy Edwards presented the first tomographic images using the Anger camera, by acquiring multiple planar images from different angles around the body and creating a three-dimensional representation. This technology, called single-photon emission computerized tomography (SPECT or SPET), is of special interest when studying complex three-dimensional anatomical structures [1, 6]. Besides static 2D and tomographic images, it is also possible to obtain dynamic, sequential images of the radiopharmaceutical's variation over time within a particular segment of the body [8].

Another indispensable nuclear-imaging method consists of positron emission tomography (PET). The distinction between SPECT and PET is based on the physical properties of the radioisotopes used for imaging. SPECT (single-photon imaging) relies on single γ-ray photon emitters. By contrast, PET uses positron emitters—radioisotopes that simultaneously emit two 511-keV photons, at approximately opposite directions. These photons are detected in the PET camera by a ring of detectors configured to detect coincidence. The registered events are then reconstructed into a three-dimensional image [5, 9].

Although PET offers some advantages over SPECT, such as improved resolution and increased quantitative capabilities, SPECT is often more practical because of its wider availability and lesser cost [3].

A typical nuclear-imaging procedure starts with the administration of the selected radiotracer, followed by image acquisition (through the detection of γ-rays, X-rays, or annihilation quanta in PET, using either a gamma camera or a PET scanner). The resulting image illustrates the tracer's location within the body [5, 10].

More recent developments in Nuclear Medicine include hybrid-imaging techniques. Hybrid imaging refers to the fusion of two (or more) imaging modalities, such as SPECT/CT, PET/CT, or PET/magnetic resonance (MR) devices. These modalities have the advantage of condensing molecular and anatomical information in a single examination, thus surpassing one major drawback of highly specific tracers: the lack of anatomical landmarks within the image [3, 4].

It should be noted that Nuclear Medicine can also operate without imagery. This can be achieved by the measurement of radioactivity in specified sites of accumulation or in biological samples following the administration of the radiopharmaceutical [1, 8].

4. Radiopharmaceuticals

The first radioactive tracer experiment was performed by George Charles de Hevesy in the 1920s. In the 1930s, Irene Curie and Frederic Joliot discovered artificial radioactivity. The discovery of the cyclotron by Ernest Lawrence opened the door for the production of radiotracers of practically every element, thus enabling investigators to design radiotracers for the study of specific biochemical processes.

The European Pharmacopoeia describes "radiopharmaceutical" as any medical product which, when ready to use, contains one or more radionuclides included for a medicinal purpose [11].

Although the field of Nuclear Medicine evolved into a more sophisticated molecular-imaging technology, the term "radiopharmaceuticals" has extended to novel radiolabeled molecular-imaging probes [1, 4].

Most radiopharmaceuticals consist of a combination of a radioactive molecule—a radionuclide—and a biologically active molecule or a drug that acts as a carrier and determines localization and biodistribution. For a few radionuclides (such as radioiodine, gallium, or thallium), the radioactive atoms themselves act as the radiopharmaceuticals [3].

The radionuclide emits radiation that is detected externally using gamma cameras or PET cameras. Certain characteristics are desirable for clinically useful radiopharmaceuticals. Radionuclide decay should result in emissions of suitable energy (100–200 keV is ideal for gamma cameras) and in sufficient abundance for external detection. Particulate radiation (e.g., beta emissions) increases the patient radiation dose, and should be reserved for therapeutic use. Effective half-life should be only long enough for the intended application (usually a few hours). The radionuclide should be carrier-free—that is, not contaminated by other stable radionuclides or other radionuclides of the same element. Technetium-99m most closely fulfills these features for the gamma camera, and fluorine-18 for PET [2, 3].

Once a decision about a suitable nuclide has been made, an appropriate agent must be selected to carry the isotope. There are many different radiopharmaceuticals available to study the different parts of the body, which can be administered by injection, ingestion, or even inhalation. They are administered in sub-pharmacological doses (<100 μg) and "trace" a particular physiological or pathological process in the body, portraying the physiology, biochemistry, or pathology, without affecting it or without causing any other physiological effect [2, 3]. Thus, with the exception of some tracers in radio-immunoscintigraphy and radiotherapy, hypersensitivity reactions against tracers are very rare, as the administered quantities are below a threshold to trigger immune response. Even in known hypersensitivity to iodinated substances (i.e., hypersensitivity against contrast media in radiology), iodine tracers can be safely used for diagnosis and therapy [1].

Understanding the mechanism and rationale for the use of each agent is critical to understanding the normal and pathological findings demonstrated scintigraphically.

http://dx.doi.org/10.5772/65708

5. Nuclear Medicine: its applications

Taking advantage of the combination of individual characteristics of the patient and molecular specificities of the disease, Nuclear Medicine aims to integrate patient- and disease-specific information [4, 8].

Apart from its major diagnostic and therapeutic roles, Nuclear Medicine is important in establishing prognosis, assessing disease progression, identifying recurrence, selecting the most effective therapy, monitoring therapy, and adapting treatment plans in response to changes in cellular activity [1, 4, 8].

Additionally, Nuclear Medicine is an important tool in the development of new targeted drugs and in the design and implementation of improved patient-tailored therapies [1, 4, 8].

5.1. Diagnosis

Nuclear Medicine dedicates primarily to the diagnosis of medical conditions. Depending on the type of examination, radiopharmaceuticals are administered in the most suitable way, for example, intravenously or orally. Afterwards, external detectors capture the radiation emitted by those radiopharmaceuticals and images are formed, showing the radiopharmaceutical uptake distribution and, subsequently, the targeted sites.

5.2. Targeted therapy

Drugs are designed to treat diseases, correcting abnormal cellular or molecular processes [4]. In theory, any highly specific imaging tracer can be used for therapy if labeled with the suitable radionuclide.

The term theranostics refers to substances that have both diagnostic and therapeutic roles. One classic example is radioiodine, used to diagnose and treat some thyroid pathologies. Theranostics has played a vital role in radiation-based therapies, especially when using targeted radiopharmaceuticals [9, 12].

Therapeutic procedures in Nuclear Medicine use high-dose, nonpenetrating radiation emitting, targeted radiopharmaceuticals. Most therapies use beta-emitters (I-131, Y-90, and Lu-177), but Auger-, Alpha-, or conversion electron emitters are also good candidates [3, 8]. The targeting ligands can also be radiolabeled with suitable positron emitters such as F-18 and Ga-68, for PET monitoring and evaluation purposes [9].

Theranostics agents play a major role in the development of radiopharmaceuticals, validating its target profile and early-disease diagnostics. They help choose the more adequate candidates and therefore are frequently used by the pharmaceutical industry [9].

5.3. Drug and formulation development and drug-regulatory affairs

Nuclear Medicine studies on drug delivery have been accepted by regulatory authorities as supporting evidence in product registration dossiers such as Investigational New Drug Applications or New Drug Applications [13].

Nuclear Medicine stimulates and supports drug development in a noninvasive way. With the radiolabeling of drug molecules, it is possible to monitor distribution, release, and kinetics, through the observation of its *in vivo* distribution and allowing the visualization of their metabolism in both target and nontarget sites [1, 13]. These studies can be performed in both animals and humans.

In drug approval, most studies are performed with new chemical entities (NCEs), because information on their metabolic outcome is required. Studies of biopharmaceuticals metabolism using radiotracers are less frequent, because it can be difficult to substitute a radiotracer for a naturally occurring stable isotope [6].

Regulatory drug-testing programs that employ radiotracers are generally classified into two groups: explorative and standard studies. Standard studies are habitually done for the majority of NCEs, with varying characteristics, depending on the drug class and specific circumstances. Explorative studies, although very important (even mandatory sometimes), are not usually required. More than 80% of all drug-safety-testing assessment programs (by the US safety assessment process) used radiotracers [14].

6. Drug delivery and Nuclear Medicine

Drugs are usually administered as pharmaceutical dosage forms. In the development of these dosage forms, it is fundamental to ensure they will perform correctly. Before the submission to the regulatory authority for approval of a new medicine, detailed testing is required. To improve therapeutic effects and minimize toxicity, it is crucial to deliver the therapeutic drugs to the right target, in the desired time, and in the precise concentration—a "magic bullet" [7, 9].

The controlled and targeted delivery of therapeutic drugs improves their bioavailability (either by preventing premature degradation or by improving uptake), maintains their concentrations within the therapeutic window (by adjusting the release rate), and reduces side effects (by targeting disease site/cells). The ability to deliver therapeutic drugs to the target, in a minimally invasive approach, has advanced considerably with the growth of molecular-imaging techniques [9].

When molecular-imaging radiotracers are part of the drug-delivery system, they enable monitoring of its *in vivo* behaviour: pharmacokinetics, distribution, release at the target site, and excretion. Some of these evaluations (such as *in vivo* fate or delivery efficiency) are not possible with a nonimage-guided approach. Another issue with nonimaging techniques is that much testing (bioavailability, therapeutic efficacy, and dose response) must be done in separate experiments, which makes for a rather expensive and stressful process [9].

The use of Nuclear Medicine imaging in the study of a drug-delivery process dates back to the late 1970s and is well established in pharmaceutical development. Understanding drug action and providing key information about the drug-delivery process through a variety of routes, Nuclear Medicine can be used in the various stages of studies [6, 9, 13]. Without radiotracers, the comprehension of numerous biochemical processes would have been tremendously difficult and, in some cases, maybe impossible. Its strength lies in the quantitative nature of the images. Only Nuclear Medicine techniques can determine the precise location of tablet disintegration in the gastrointestinal (GI) tract, the depth of penetration of a nebulized solution in the lungs, or for how long does the formulation stay in the cornea [6, 9, 13].

In image-guided drug delivery assessment, the image techniques are used for determining disease location, drug-targeting levels and localization, and release kinetics (before and during treatment). The type and stability of the labeling will depend upon whether the study is meant to examine release, deposition, retention/dispersion, or is being used to monitor the effects of physiological process [13, 15].

The majority of studies have evaluated gastrointestinal, pulmonary, and nasal drug delivery, but ophthalmic, buccal, rectal, vaginal, and parenteral routes have also been subject of research [6].

The required quantity of radiotracer in a drug formulation is very small and does not commit with the performance of the delivery system. Radiolabeling must reveal high *in vitro* and *in vivo* stability and can be performed in two different ways. The radiolabeled compound can be directly incorporated into the preparation, or a dosage form that contains a nonradioactive tracer can be neutron-activated. The latter is advantageous in extensive or complicated delivery systems, and also has the advantage of the dosage formulation being manufactured and produced under normal conditions [7, 9]. Still, Nuclear Medicine imaging of drug-delivery processes involves several challenges and is affected by numerous factors such as target expression, *in vivo* availability of the receptor, type of drug, enhanced permeability and retention effect, tracer protein dose, and timing of imaging [9].

Once administered, the radiolabeled compound will be monitored *in vivo* over a period of time (depending on its half-life), using appropriate image equipment: gamma-scintigraphy or PET. It is then crucial to choose the most suitable radioisotopes, with fitting half-lives to pair with the pharmacokinetics of their drug carriers, and the most adequate imaging system [6, 9, 13].

In the last decades, most studies used gamma-scintigraphy and Tc-99m-labeled radiopharmaceuticals containing chelating agents (such as diethylene-triamine-pentaacetic acid (DTPA)), colloids (such as sulfur colloid), diphosphonates (such as hydroxymethane diphosphonate (HDP)), cells and blood elements, and cellulose macromolecules [7, 13].

More recently, the use of PET is increasing, including in drug-delivery development studies. An important attribute of PET studies is that some of the radioactive atoms available include radioisotopes of carbon, nitrogen, and fluorine. This makes it possible to synthesize PET radiotracers with the same chemical structure as the unlabeled molecules, without altering their biological function [9, 13].

Unlike radiological imaging, Nuclear Medicine allows serial images to be obtained without submitting the subjects to higher radiation burdens, and radioactive concerns are neglected. Besides the reliability and reproducibility of Nuclear Medicine studies on the nature and characteristics of products, they may also be performed in the groups of patients intended to receive the dosage forms therapeutically, which is important since the presence of pathology can have significant impact on physiology [13].

It is well established that diseases alter physiological processes, and subsequently biodistribution of drug formulations. Thus, studies in humans are the most relevant and Nuclear Medicine imaging probably represents the only technique available that allows the quantification of drug release and pharmacokinetics in specific groups, namely patients with diseases [13]. This know-how has the potential for patient selection for targeted therapy and for the monitoring of therapeutic response after the drug is delivered [9].

Targeted therapy involves the integration of multidisciplinary fields such as cell and molecular biology, chemistry, physics, and so on. Significant advances in the field have been attributed to the progress in nanotechnology, with the development of nanosized, multifunctional drug-delivery platforms. For example, a single platform can be used to detect, treat, and monitor treatment response in tumors. These systems present several advantages, including minimal clearance by the immune system, prolonged circulating times, attachment to suitable vectors (peptides, proteins, antibodies, etc.) and targeting of specific receptors, and improved treatment effects by shielding entrapped drugs from degradation [9].

For example, stimulus-responsive polymeric nanomaterials can be synthesized to mimic the behavior of biological molecules, minimizing side effects and maximizing predictability. Another example, the liposomal carriers (the first and most extensive studied drug-delivery carriers), is used in the delivery of anticancer drugs, antineoplastic agents, antimicrobial compounds, immunomodulators, anti-inflammatory agents, cardiovascular drugs, and so on. Some other nanosized drug-delivery systems that have also been developed for molecular-imaging purposes are metallic nanoparticles, oxide nanoparticles, polymeric nanoparticles, and carbon nanostructures [9].

The major goal of molecular imaging is to maximize therapy effect in diseased tissues, and reduce systemic effects and toxicity as much as possible [9].

6.1. Gastrointestinal tract studies

Despite the vast diversity of new drug-delivery systems, oral administration is still preferred.

Most commonly, oral-dosage forms immediately release in the stomach, but the use of more sophisticated, modified release systems is increasing and requires new methods of evaluation. Furthermore, regulatory authorities require evaluation of the *in vivo* performance of new oral formulations.

Nuclear Medicine imaging is one of the most popular methods to investigate those GI release systems, because pharmacokinetic measurements are often unreliable. Its combination with pharmacokinetic studies provides accurate data about transit, absorption, and release performance of oral-dosage formulations [7].

Nuclear Medicine imaging provides information, from both control and patient groups, on swallowing dynamics of tablet and capsule formulations, disintegration of immediate release formulations, gastric emptying and gastroesophageal reflux, release of enteric-coated formulations, GI transit times, the effect of formulation size on GI delivery, visualization of targeted release or delivery to the colon, the effects of time of dosing on delivery, local permeability

http://dx.doi.org/10.5772/65708

within the colon, disintegration characteristics likely to influence drug absorption, and residence time of the material within the colon [7, 9].

GI nuclear studies often require both solid- and liquid-phase markers, there being two conventional approaches for the labeling of the oral-dosage forms. One method involves incorporating a nonabsorbable chelate of the radioactive isotope (e.g., DTPA-Tc-99m). The other incorporating a radiolabeled ion-exchange resin, which has the advantage of giving information about the *in vivo* position of the radiolabeled drug, because the resin remains within the device [7].

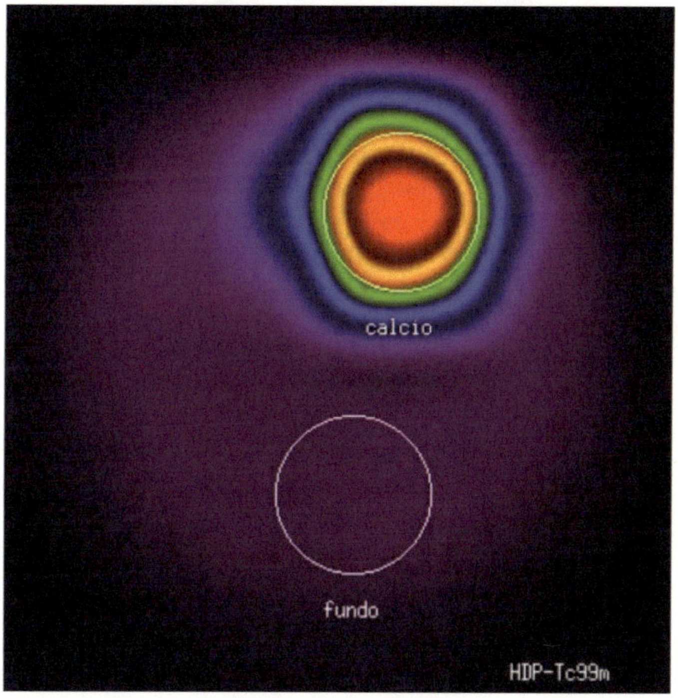

Figure 1. *In vitro* radiolabeling and evaluation of the drug-delivery system.

In two different studies aimed at evaluating the gastroretentive behavior of pharmaceutical dosage forms, Barata et al. used Tc-99m-HDP to label HMPC tablets supplemented with calcium phosphate. The radiolabeling process consisted in soaking the tablet in a Tc-99m-HDP and NaCl 0.9% solution, with activity counts of 400–600 millicuries. The addition of calcium to the systems did not affect drug release, but significantly increased the binding of the radiopharmaceutical to the dosage form. In fact, the dosage form remained integer and well radiolabeled for a period of over 4 h, which was sufficient to study the gastroretentive pattern of the produced tablets. This proved to be an easy and reproducible method of extemporaneously radiolabeling tablets produced outside Nuclear Medicine Department facilities, solving radiation-related transportation problems (see **Figure 1**).

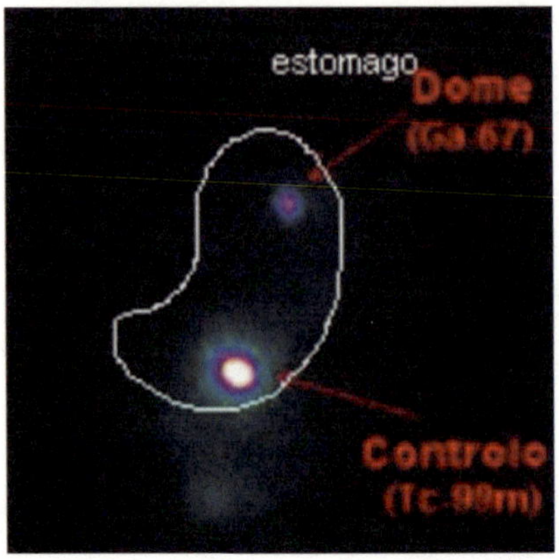

Figure 2. *In vivo* analysis of the drug-delivery system floating behavior.

For the floating-device study, a non-floating tablet was labeled with Tc-99m-HDP, while the floating pharmaceutical dosage form was labeled with Ga-68 (gallium-68), using the same soaking method. Despite not as effective as Tc-99m-HDP labeling, Ga-68 labeling was enough to allow a clear visualization of the system. The physical properties of the two radiopharmaceuticals (different energy photons) enabled the simultaneous identifying of each system over time: initially, both in the stomach (floating in the upper part of the stomach or staying in the antrum), then, the effective gastroretention of the floating device for over 4 h (see **Figure 2**).

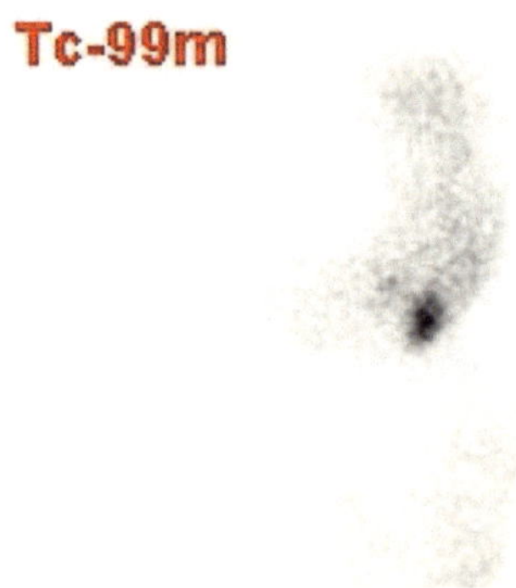

Figure 3. *In vivo* analysis of the drug-delivery system gastroretentive behavior.

In the other study, aiming to demonstrate the gastroretentive efficacy of high-density tablets, a similar process was used to radiolabel the produced tablets. Again, it was possible to see the *in vivo* positioning of the pharmaceutical dosage form and confirm that the high-density controlled release strategy is effective for delivering drugs with a narrow upper GI absorption window (see **Figure 3**).

These examples prove that incorporating gamma-emitting radionuclides into a delivery device or formulation provides an appropriate, simple method of observing the transit and residence within the GI tract—of particular interest in determining the time and site of release of delayed release formulations.

6.2. Other system studies

Both SPECT and PET imaging play an increasing role in the development of new targeted drug-delivery systems [13].

Nuclear Medicine is being used to surpass the severe systemic toxicity of anticancer drugs, which are usually more effective in high doses. Additionally, numerous conventional therapeutic agents repeatedly fail to reach their target, rendering them ineffective. The ideal drug should be specific for the cancer cell and devoid of systemic effects. For these reasons, the ideal drug-delivery system is aimed, and Nuclear Medicine, with all its already-known advantages, plays an important role in this area [9, 16].

PET image-guided drug delivery allows for the treatment of a variety of diseases with minimal systemic involvement (sparing normal cells), while monitoring its efficacy.

In cancer-targeted treatment, chemotherapeutic drugs can be loaded onto multifunctional drug carriers (such as liposomes, micelles, and nanoparticles) and coupled with several targeting ligands (such as monoclonal antibodies, peptides, and antibody fragments). Carriers are multifunctional and may also carry PET radiopharmaceuticals for diagnostic purposes. These systems are important examples of theranostics. One example is the streptavidin/biotin interaction that is used for binding numerous carriers to targeting proteins and antibodies.

In another approach, therapeutic radionuclides are conjugated with targeting ligands (by means of bifunctional-linking strategies), without any image-enabling radionuclide. PET imaging for the diagnosis or monitoring of therapeutic response is carried out separately, by conjugation of the targeting ligands with suitable PET radioisotopes [9].

Investigation-wise, PET allows the *in vivo* quantification and drug distribution, determining its extraction fraction and washout from different organs/systems.

PET imaging allows the study of the first-pass liver elimination of a drug, a fundamental knowledge, since first-pass metabolism excludes oral delivery of several drug molecules and compounds.

PET studies are also useful in the understanding of the brain and of several neurological conditions, including anxiety and depression [13]. In Parkinson's and Alzheimer's diseases, the *in vivo* study of neuroreceptors binding is fundamental for the drug-design process (ex. enzyme/prodrug-based delivery approach with 18F for Parkinson's disease) [9, 13].

7. Conclusion

Nuclear Medicine is a very promising field and will surely increase its relevance on diagnostics and therapeutics in the near future. Also within the field of drug development and drug-delivery systems research, it is expected to demonstrate an ever-increasing applicability and importance. The advent of new and more complex drugs, combined with more ingenious and technological delivery systems, will call for a more detailed and effective *in vivo* studies during the development and regulatory phases of the research and marketing authorization process. Radiopharmaceuticals and Nuclear Medicine will therefore be predictably ever more used with the purpose of obtaining better, safer, and more reliable drug-delivery systems.

Author details

Ana Rita Fernandes[1], Ana Oliveira[1], Jorge Pereira[1] and Pedro Silva Coelho[2*]

*Address all correspondence to: pbarata@ufp.edu.pt

1 Nuclear Medicine Department, São João Hospital Center, Porto, Portugal

2 Faculty of Health Sciences, University Fernando Pessoa, Porto, Portugal

References

[1] Leitha T. Nuclear Medicine: Proof of principle for targeted drugs in diagnosis and therapy. Current Pharmaceutical Design. 2009;15:173–187. DOI: 10.2174/138161209787002898

[2] Society of Nuclear Medicine [Internet]. Available from: http://interactive.snm.org/docs/whatisnucmed2.pdf and http://www.snmmi.org/AboutSNMMI/Content.aspx?ItemNumber=6433 [Accessed: 2016.05.23]

[3] Ziessman HA, O'Malley JP, Thrall JH. Nuclear Medicine: The Requisites. 4th ed. Philadelphia, PA: Elsevier; 2013. 466 p. DOI: 10.1148/radiol.2223012567.

[4] Clanton J, Sandler MP. Molecular imaging radiopharmaceuticals for PET and SPECT. Journal of Nuclear Medicine. 2010;51:660–661. DOI: 10.2967/jnumed.109.072645

[5] Kim EE, Lee D, Tateishi U, Baum RP. Handbook of Nuclear Medicine and Molecular Imaging—Principles and Clinical Applications. 2nd ed. World Scientific Publishing Co. Pte. Ltd., 2012. 472 p. ISBN: 9789814366236

[6] Lappin G, Temple S. Radiotracers in Drug Development. Taylor & Francis, 2006. 320 p. ISBN: 9780849333477

[7] Wilding IR, Coupe AJ, Davis SS. The role of γ-scintigraphy in oral drug delivery. Advanced Drug Delivery Reviews. 2001;46:103–124. DOI: 10.1016/S0169-409X(00)00135-6.

[8] Calahan RJ. et al. Society of nuclear medicine procedure guideline for the use of radiopharmaceuticals 4.0. Journal of Nuclear Medicine Technology. 2007;35(4) 272–275. DOI: 10.2967/jnmt.107.044156.

[9] Chakravarty R, Hong H, Cai W. Positron emission tomography image-guided drug delivery: Current status and future perspectives. Molecular Pharmaceutics. 2014; 11(11):3777–3797. DOI: 10.1021/mp500173s

[10] Baert AL, Sartor K, Schiepers C. Diagnostic Nuclear Medicine. 2nd Revised Edition. Springer-Verlag, Berlin Heidelberg, 2006. 355 p. DOI: 10.1007/3-540-30005-8

[11] European Pharmacopoeia. 8th ed. EDQM, 01/2014., 2016. ISBN-13:9789287175274

[12] MacKay JA, Li Z. Theranostic agents that co-deliver therapeutic and imaging agents? Advanced Drug Delivery Reviews. 2010;62(11):1003–1004. DOI: 10.1016/j.addr.2010.10.001

[13] Malcolm F, Alan CP. The role of gamma scintigraphy in the study of drug delivery. Correspondence Continuing Education Courses for Nuclear Pharmacists and Nuclear Medicine Professional. 2003;X(N° 3 and 4):1–76.

[14] Roberts D, Lockley R. Radiosynthesis: A vital role supporting drug development. Drug Discovery World, Fall, 2004, pp. 59–62.

[15] Hatefi A, Minko T. Advances in image-guided drug delivery. Drug Delivery and Translational Research. 2012;2:1–2. DOI: 10.1007/s13346-011-0057-8.

[16] Haley B, Frenkel E. Nanoparticles for drug delivery in cancer treatment. Urologic Oncology. 2008;26(1):57–64. DOI: 10.1016/j.urolonc.2007.03.015.